MW01231454

Facts About AIDS

A GUIDE FOR HEALTH CARE PROVIDERS

Facts About AIDS

A GUIDE
FOR HEALTH CARE PROVIDERS

Sue Perdew, RN, PhD
Chairperson and Associate Professor

Department of Nursing
Marywood College
Scranton, Pennsylvania

J. B. Lippincott Company
Philadelphia
Grand Rapids   New York   St. Louis
San Francisco   London   Sydney   Tokyo

Acquiring Editor: Patricia Cleary
Sponsoring Editor: Donna L. Hilton
Manuscript Editor: Terry Schutz
Production Manager: Janet Greenwood
Production: Publishers' WorkGroup
Compositor: Publications Development Co.
Printer/Binder: R. R. Donnelley & Sons

6 5 4 3 2 1

Library of Congress Cataloging in Publication Data

Perdew, Sue.
    Facts about AIDS : a guide for health care providers / Sue Perdew.
      p. cm.
    Bibliography: p.
    Includes index.
    ISBN 0-397-54768-4
    1. AIDS (Disease) 2. AIDS (Disease)—Prevention. 3. Medical
personnel—Health and hygiene. I. Title.
    [DNLM: 1. Acquired Immunodeficiency Syndrome—prevention &
control. 2. Acquired Immunodeficiency Syndrome—nursing. WD 308
P433f]
    RC607.A26P45 1990
    616.97'92—dc20
    DNLM/DLC
    for Library of Congress   89-12631
                                                                    CIP

Any procedure or practice described in this book should be applied by the
health-care practitioner under appropriate supervision in accordance with
professional standards of care used with regard to the unique circumstances that apply in each practice situation. Care has been taken to confirm the accuracy of information presented and to describe generally
accepted practices. However, the authors, editors and publisher cannot accept any responsibility for errors or omissions or for consequences from
application of the information in this book and make no warranty, express
or implied, with respect to the contents of the book.

Every effort has been made to ensure drug selections and dosages are in
accordance with current recommendations and practice. Because of ongoing research, changes in government regulations and the constant flow
of information on drug therapy, reactions and interactions, the reader is
cautioned to check the package insert for each drug for indications,
dosages, warnings and precautions, particularly if the drug is new or
infrequently used.

For Desi

with deepest respect,
affection, and hope
for a brighter tomorrow

PREFACE

With the advent of acquired immunodeficiency syndrome (AIDS), health care has changed. The public, previously confident and perhaps complacent about the ability of modern medicine to treat illness, has had a rude awakening; deadly new diseases baffle the scientific community and instill fear in it as well as in the public—fear of the diseases and also of the sick people who may transmit them. Nurses and other direct care providers generally want to provide good care to all patients, but sometimes fear gets in the way. The term *health care provider* in this book broadly identifies any person who gives hands-on care to ill people. Health care providers may be employed to provide care, or they may be volunteers. They may be trained as nurses or nursing assistants, or they may have very little training.

This book presents basic information about AIDS to health care providers in order to enable them to treat AIDS patients and others well and without undue risk. Information will be limited to what providers need in order to understand current thinking about the disease, current recommendations of health care authorities for preventing the disease, and current issues related to AIDS and human immunodeficiency virus (HIV) infection. Excellent texts exist on providing care to AIDS patients; this book will not address that subject except in the most general way.

Chapter 1 presents basic information about HIV, the virus that causes AIDS. It covers the immune system, diagnosis, transmission, and prevention. Chapter 2 provides detailed information on preventing transmission of disease in the settings in which people commonly provide health care. The tests used to identify the presence of the virus in people are discussed in Chapter 3. Societal, legal, and ethical issues that arise from this epidemic are considered in

Chapter 4. Chapter 5 identifies the various U.S. government agencies and divisions responsible for dealing with the epidemic and provides a list of community resources to use in addressing the complex problems brought about by the epidemic. Chapter 6 provides an explanation of employers' obligations toward health care providers and patients, and Chapter 7 answers questions commonly asked of and by health care providers. A glossary is provided to assist the reader.

While the chapters may be read in any order, topics are presented in a logical sequence. Information about the virus and the immune system and about HIV infection and AIDS is followed by information on protecting yourself. Some readers will be satisfied with just this much information. Readers interested in the broader issues mentioned above, however, should find Chapters 3 through 6 useful. The final chapter, Questions and Answers, is a quick review in a different format of the most pertinent information; it should help the provider to present material to others—colleagues, patients, family, the public.

While I have tried to provide information that is up to date, research on AIDS advances rapidly, as does information about related legal, ethical, and societal issues. To be truly well informed and protected, the reader must be always alert to new information regarding HIV infection.

SUE PERDEW, RN, PhD

ACKNOWLEDGMENTS

I would like to thank Dr. Francis X. Lobo, Professor of Biology at Marywood College, Scranton, Pennsylvania, for his invaluable assistance in the preparation of Chapter 1. Colleagues who assisted in reviewing sections of the book include Patricia Yanul, RN, Esterina Bevilaqua, RN, Ann St. Ledger, RN, and Joe Kishel, RN. Charlotte Woodward helped me learn to use the word processor.

I would like to thank, also, the nursing staff in the Renal Dialysis Unit at Moses Taylor Hospital, Scranton. The nursing staff at Moses Taylor taught me a lot through their professional and thoughtful care of several friends who suffered from AIDS.

My husband, Paul Perdew, read and reviewed sections, encouraged me to think more logically, and gave me hugs PRN.

CONTENTS

Facts About AIDS

A GUIDE FOR HEALTH CARE PROVIDERS

1

HIV INFECTION: HISTORY, DIAGNOSIS, TRANSMISSION, AND PREVENTION

This chapter discusses the history and biology of the human immunodeficiency virus (HIV) infection and various aspects of acquired immunodeficiency syndrome (AIDS) as this disease is presently seen in the United States. It also considers transmission of HIV and methods that may be used to prevent infection.

HISTORY

Through recorded history certain diseases have been associated with dread and panic: leprosy, plague, polio, and syphilis. There are distinct similarities between public reaction to venereal disease in the early 1900s and reaction to AIDS today: the pervasive fear of contagion; concerns about casual transmission; stigmatization of infected persons; and conflicts between protecting public health and ensuring civil liberties (Brandt, 1987).

AIDS and the fear which some have termed "afrAIDS" (acute fear regarding AIDS) touch upon the deepest feelings of all of us—feelings about security, morality, death, and disfigurement. Following a proud tradition, today's health care providers have an unusual opportunity to serve by presenting a united, rational perspective to their patients and to the public.

BIOLOGY OF HIV INFECTION

AIDS and the conditions associated with it are caused by HIV, the human immunodeficiency virus. Normally a person's body provides protection from viruses and other

1

foreign invaders through a complex process known as the immune response.

The Immune Response

When pathogens—disease-bearing organisms—enter the body, they are literally eaten up in the process of phagocytosis by white blood cells called macrophages. Macrophages (the name loosely translated means "big eater") are the body's scavengers; they clean up dead cells and foreign material and are the main actors fighting disease in the bloodstream.

Several other white blood cells are also important to the immune response; these include T lymphocytes and B lymphocytes. Two types of T lymphocytes that are especially important are T helper and T killer cells.

Antigen-Antibody Reaction

In the process of ingesting foreign cells, the macrophage takes the unique protein coat of the foreigner and displays a piece on its own surface. This piece of protein, called an *antigen,* elicits an immune response that produces antibodies designed specifically to destroy or inactivate the intruder.

Displayed on the surface of a macrophage, the antigen acts as a "battle call" to muster the body's attack forces. At the center of this effort is the T helper cell (T4 lymphocyte). A special few of these helpers lock onto the antigen, which is not itself infectious, because it is only a small part of the foreign cell. After being "sensitized" to the particular antigen, the T helper is ready to send out several chemical signals to begin an attack upon the pathogen.

To mediate, or control, the immune response having to do with specific cells, the T helper does three things.

- The T helper sends out chemicals that increase the production of the special type of T helper that matches the protein coat of the foreigner.
- The T helper sends a chemical message to the spleen and lymph nodes to modify some cells to carry out certain

additional functions. Some of the cells modified in this process are called T killer cells. Among other actions, these T killers destroy viruses that reproduce inside other cells by puncturing the cell membrane of the host cell and allowing the contents of the cell, including the viruses, to spill out into the bloodstream, where they can be engulfed by macrophages.

The spleen and lymph nodes have a limited supply of T cells, which have been present since early childhood and are not replenished. Although originally large in number, they can be used up, leaving the body without one of its greatest sources of protection.

• Finally, through chemical messages, the T helper communicates with B lymphocytes in the spleen and lymph nodes. These B lymphocytes make the antibodies that circulate in the body's fluids and latch onto the projections of the invader so that it cannot enter a body cell. The invader cell subsequently dies without multiplying.

There are limits to the protection that antibodies provide against foreign invaders. In the first place, an antibody response takes weeks or months to achieve its maximum strength. Also, like macrophages, antibodies can only attack viruses that are free-floating in the fluids of the body. And, since each antibody is specific for only one antigen, if a virus alters its protein coat even slightly, the antibody may not recognize it. Many viruses, including HIV, alter their protein coats, even within one person's body, making it possible to be infected with several subtypes of the virus at the same time.

Life Cycle of Viruses

Viruses are composed of nucleic acid, either DNA or RNA, surrounded by a protein coat called a capsid. See Figure 1–1. Viruses cannot live on their own but require a host for survival and multiplication. Viral hosts may be plants, animals, bacteria, protozoa, fungi, and algae. These parasites are so small that a special electron microscope is required to "see" them.

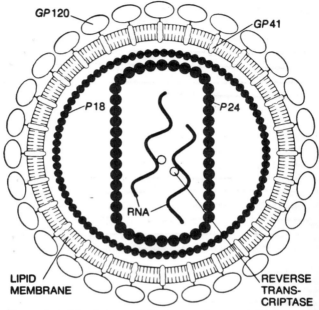

Figure 1–1. Morphology of the human immunodeficiency virus (HIV). HTLV-III virion, or virus particle, is a sphere that is roughly 1,000 angstrom units (one ten-thousandth of a millimeter) across. The particle is covered by a membrane, made up of two layers of lipid (fatty) material, that is derived from the outer membrane of the host cell. Studding the membrane are glycoproteins (proteins with sugar chains attached). Each glycoprotein has two components: *gp*41 spans the membrane and *gp*120 extends beyond it. The membrane-and-protein envelope covers a core made up of proteins designated *p*24 and *p*18. The viral RNA is carried in the core, along with several copies of the enzyme reverse transcriptase, which catalyzes the assembly of the viral DNA. Adapted from an illustration by George V. Kelvin, Science Graphics, 6 Devon Road, Greatneck, New York, 11023. From The AIDS virus by Robert Gallo. *Scientific American,* 1987, Jan., 256(1): 48.

A virus may begin reproducing itself immediately upon entering a host cell, or it may "hide" for a short or long period of time. A virus that is in hiding is said to be "latent." HIV is such a virus.

When HIV (floating freely or hiding within a cell) in the blood, semen, or vaginal fluid of an infected person enters the blood of an uninfected person, the virus is either attacked by a macrophage, starting the process described above, or is admitted through the protein coat of a T helper cell with glycoprotein matching its own.

Now incorporated into the genetic material of the host cell, HIV waits for some stimulus—not presently known—to begin to multiply. An infected person can pass the virus to other people through sperm, blood, or vaginal fluid, even though the HIV-infected person is not sick. The especially devastating effect of HIV is related to the fact that the cell used by the virus to reproduce is the very cell the body needs to direct an attack on the virus—the T helper cell.

So many HIVs are produced within an activated T helper cell that they burst out of the cell membrane, killing the cell. These viruses, now floating freely in the blood, infect other T helpers, eventually killing them. Since the body has only a limited supply of T cells, the death of large numbers of these protectors leaves the infected person open to attack from pathogens that, in a healthy person, are killed under the direction of T helper cells.

Human Immunodeficiency Virus (HIV) in the Body

HIVs floating freely in the blood stimulate B lymphocytes to start producing antibodies to HIV. Unfortunately, by the time enough antibodies to HIV are produced to mount an effective attack, the viruses have invaded other cells where they are safe from the attacking antibodies.

Another chemical message, or signal, stimulates formation of T killer cells, which multiply and attack the cells breeding the HIV. Thus, T helpers with HIV are killed by the very T killer cells they have called to attack the enemy.

Progress of Infection

Even before an infected person has symptoms of HIV infection, the progress of the infection can be detected by determining, through blood tests, the numbers and ratios of certain critical white blood cells (see Figure 1–2).

Control of Viral Diseases

Control of disease is brought about by prevention or by treatment; prevention, or *prophylaxis*, is obviously preferable to treatment. Vaccination against viral disease can be a very effective method of prevention, as has been shown in the cases of smallpox, measles, mumps, influenza, hepatitis B, poliomyelitis, rabies, and yellow fever. However, in spite of intense, global efforts to develop a vaccine for HIV, success in this endeavor is many years away.

DIAGNOSIS OF AIDS AND HIV INFECTION

A Disease by Definition

A diagnosis of AIDS is unlike diagnoses of most other major life-threatening illnesses. While many cancers can be diagnosed by looking at cells under a microscope, and other diseases may be diagnosed by laboratory tests or X-rays, AIDS is a disease *by definition*. That is, AIDS is a combination of signs and symptoms (a syndrome).

AIDS is an acquired illness of the immune system which reduces the body's ability to fight specific types of infections and cancers. AIDS is caused by the human immunodeficiency virus (HIV) and is transmitted through intimate sexual contact, in particular anal and vaginal intercourse, or through direct exposure to infected blood. HIV may also be transmitted from an infected pregnant woman to her fetus before or during birth, or to her infant through infected breast milk. Persons who are diagnosed as having AIDS are HIV positive and have developed one or more unusual opportunistic bacterial, fungal, or viral infections

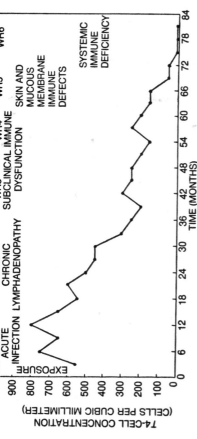

Figure 1–2. Progression of immune dysfunction over time. Decline in T4 cell count (rounded to the nearest 50) was tracked in the blood of a young man whose disease followed a typical course. About three months after sexual exposure to HIV the patient tested positive for the virus; his T4 cell count dropped and then rebounded, presumably because his immune system temporarily controlled the infection. He developed chronic lymphadenopathy at nine months and, at 51 months, after a long, slow decline in his T4 cell count (by 36 months it was chronically below 400), exhibited chronic, subtle abnormalities of delayed hypersensitivity. He displayed persistent anergy (the complete absence of delayed hypersensitivity) at 63 months but had no overt symptoms of infection until about 68 months, when he developed thrush and oral hairy leukoplakia, a tongue infection. Less than a year later he was besieged by opportunistic infections, including cytomegalovirus infection, which made him blind. He died at 83 months. Illustration by Ian Worpole. From HIV infection: The clinical picture, by Robert R. Redfield and Donald S. Burke. Copyright 1988 by Scientific American, Inc., *Scientific American*, 1988 Oct; 259(4): 94. All rights reserved.

or rare cancers. All cases of AIDS must be reported to the Centers for Disease Control (CDC).

The CDC currently classifies AIDS-related infection in adults according to whether specific indicator diseases are present in an individual and whether there is laboratory evidence (antibody or other test) of HIV infection (Centers for Disease Control, 1987).

Aspects (Signs) of the Disease

As with other diseases, AIDS presents certain *signs* and *symptoms* in a person. A *sign* of disease is evidence that can be verified objectively. Some signs of AIDS are a positive HIV antibody test, a diagnosed opportunistic disease, an alteration in the T4 lymphocyte count, enlarged lymph nodes, loss of weight, and persistent diarrhea.

A *symptom* of a disease is a sensation experienced by the patient. The symptoms of AIDS and of some other HIV conditions include shortness of breath, fatigue, loss of memory, and loss of appetite. They are related to the specific opportunistic infections the patient contracts and, in some instances, quite possibly to the direct destruction of cells by the virus.

The Potential to Harm

AIDS is most certainly a deadly disease. Of persons officially diagnosed as having AIDS for three years or longer, more than eighty percent have died (Rowe & Ryan, 1987). Although the length of survival after diagnosis varies according to the specific infections a person has, and according to the age, sex, and ethnic background of the patient, the disease is most often fatal within two to three years of diagnosis.

In addition to people who have symptoms of disease, HIV profoundly affects those who have tested positive for the antibody but have no symptoms. Such individuals are advised to abstain from sexual intercourse or to modify risky sexual practices in order to protect themselves and to

avoid infecting others. Women must be informed of the
risk of bearing infected children. An infected person may
not be able to work in a chosen field or may be denied
health and life insurance.

Categories of Disease

The public, the press, and the media have generally come
to know three categories of AIDS-related infection: (1) HIV
infection without symptoms; (2) AIDS-related complex
(ARC); (3) AIDS (the disease). The ARC category lacks a
commonly accepted definition and is not used by the CDC.
The public, however, understands this category as including
those people who are infected with HIV and have symptoms
but in whom AIDS has not been diagnosed.

Thinking of HIV-infected people in these categories em-
phasizes how large the pool of infected and infectious people is. This concept may motivate some people to avoid
risky sexual practices and IV drug injection. On the other
hand, grouping people in this way may mask the progressive aspects of the illness and may deny some HIV-infected
people access to public funds for which eligibility is arbi-
trarily limited.

Current CDC Categories

The CDC issues a weekly update, the *AIDS Weekly
Surveillance Report,* which is sent free of charge to any individual or organization requesting it. In this report, U.S. occurrences of AIDS reported to CDC are grouped into the
following transmission categories:

Adults/adolescents

- Homosexual or bisexual male
- Intravenous (IV) drug abuser
- Homosexual male, IV drug abuser
- Hemophilia or other coagulation disorder
- Heterosexual person
- Transfusion of blood or blood components
- Undetermined

Children

- Hemophilia or other coagulation disorder
- Parent with or at risk of AIDS
- Transfusion of blood or blood components
- Undetermined

Patients are further categorized by race and ethnic group, by state of residence, by date of diagnosis, and by major risk factor. Deaths are reported by date of AIDS diagnosis and by opportunistic disease category. Age at diagnosis is reported by racial and ethnic group.

The Pyramid of Disease Progression

Figure 1–3 presents a pyramid of disease progression. It is not known what proportion of HIV-infected persons will progress to full-blown AIDS, but available data indicate that more than half of those who carry the virus develop AIDS within ten years of infection, and studies have suggested that most carriers will become ill (Altman, 1989).

Not Infected

Persons not infected, fortunately including most of the population, need a range of educational services to assist them in prevention. Those presently in greatest need of prevention are sexually active adults and intravenous drug users. Also at high risk for infection are young people who are becoming sexually active and those who may start to experiment with drugs.

HIV-Positive Status

HIV-positive status designates people with initial infection, asymptomatic infection, infection with symptoms (generalized lymph node enlargement and ARC), and full-blown AIDS. People who are infected with HIV have a variety of health care needs.

Initial Infection. While the body always responds to infection in some way, the infected person may not notice or recognize this response. Many people report no symptoms

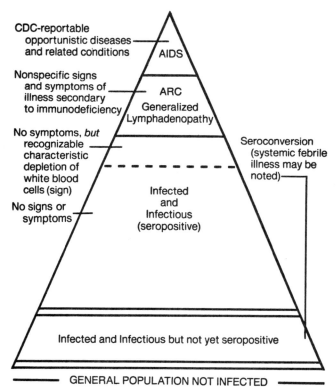

Figure 1-3. The pyramid of disease progression in a population.

in the initial phase of HIV infection. If symptoms are noted, they generally occur within two to three weeks of exposure to the virus and may include rash, fever, fatigue, and sore throat. Within a few weeks these symptoms disappear without treatment.

Asymptomatic Infection.   In August 1987, the CDC estimated that one to one and a half million people in the United States were infected with HIV (Centers for Disease Control, 1987). This estimate has not been revised. The vast majority of these people have no symptoms and may be unaware of their infected and infectious status. The presence of this large group of persons in our midst makes it necessary to treat all blood as if it is infected.

AIDS-Related Complex (ARC).   Once a person who is infected with HIV begins to have signs or symptoms brought about by a depressed immune system, he or she may be said to have the condition known as AIDS-related complex (ARC). One of the first signs of a depressed immune system is a generalized enlargement or tenderness in the lymph nodes. Persistent generalized lymphadenopathy (GLA) is brought about by increased effort of the lymph nodes to supply the body with lymphocytes to fight the enemy virus.

The person with ARC has signs and symptoms like those of many other diseases (fatigue, shortness of breath, cough, night sweats, weight loss, persistent diarrhea, rash, sores in the mouth). Lymph nodes in the neck, armpits, and groin may be enlarged. Signs and symptoms may include any or all of those listed below for AIDS, except that the person with ARC has not yet had one of the specific opportunistic infections by which AIDS is officially diagnosed. Symptoms of ARC may range from the merely annoying to conditions that make work and everyday activities impossible.

After acute episodes, the person with ARC needs evaluation by a home care nurse. Some attendant care may be needed, along with evaluation by a physician, pharmacist, physical therapist, and dietitian. Stress management related to life-threatening illness may require the assistance of a psychologist or counselor. On an intermittent basis skilled nurses will be needed to provide and to supervise care (Sedaka & O'Reilly, 1986).

The HIV-positive person, with or without symptoms, is likely to benefit by referral to community services that will help with stress management and education. People with symptoms will need support for everyday activities that can no longer be managed alone. These may include shopping, cooking, managing finances, and maintaining social relationships.

Contact with the medical community must be maintained. In this way new information about treatments and methods to enhance the immune system may be used as they become available.

Full-Blown AIDS. People who are specifically diagnosed as having AIDS are generally very sick, although at times they may feel well enough to carry on some everyday activities. These people may be homebound and increasingly unable to care for themselves. They may have decreased or greatly curtailed their outside social activities and their gainful employment. In addition, they may be depressed or have symptoms of dementia or other symptoms of central nervous system involvement.

Symptoms of AIDS include:

- Loss of appetite and unexplained weight loss of more than 10 pounds in 2 months
- Swollen glands in the neck, armpits, or groin
- Leg weakness or pain
- Unexplained fever lasting more than a week
- Night sweating, often profuse
- Persistent unexplained diarrhea
- Dry cough
- White spots or unusual blemishes in the mouth and throat (candidiasis)
- Painful blisters along the course of a nerve (shingles)
- Painless purple spots on the skin
- Progressive mental deterioration
- Loss of vision and hearing

Persons with AIDS need evaluation and consistent help from a physician, pharmacist, and dietitian. For many hours each day or possibly around the clock, they will need care from someone with knowledge or experience with AIDS prognosis and treatment. Professional nursing services will be needed to plan and supervise care and to administer intravenous drugs, fluids, and nutritional supplements. Certified home health aides may be used in the states that recognize them. The patient may be cared for in a hospital, in a hospice, or at home.

Common Opportunistic Diseases
in Persons with AIDS

The CDC has identified a list of diseases that are indicative of AIDS. These include candidiasis of the esophagus, cytomegalovirus retinitis, mycobacterioses, Kaposi's sarcoma, *Pneumocystis carinii* pneumonia, and toxoplasmosis of the brain (Centers for Disease Control, 1987). Other diseases that have become important in persons with HIV infection are cryptosporidiosis and cryptococcosis. The causes, symptoms, and treatments of these infections are briefly described below. For those interested in the nursing care of patients with these and other disorders associated with HIV infection, an excellent text is Lewis's *Nursing Care of the Person with AIDS/ARC* (Lewis, 1988).

Candidiasis Esophagitis

Candidiasis of the esophagus is caused by a yeastlike fungus, *Candida albicans*. The patient complains of pain behind the sternum on swallowing. White patches or plaques on a reddened base appearing in the mouth cannot be removed by scraping. The disease is treated with nystatin in oral suspension or with clotrimazole troche (lozenge). Both medications leave an odd taste in the mouth and may contribute to anorexia, nausea, and vomiting.

Cytomegalovirus (CMV)

CMV is a common herpes virus that causes very few problems in a person with a healthy immune system. In patients with HIV infection, however, the virus may cause blindness, pneumonia, intestinal inflammation, and inflammation and ulceration of the esophagus. CMV has also been associated with serious fetal abnormalities in the absence of HIV infection. Present treatment is limited to intravenous administration of the antiviral DHPG (ganciclovir), which has proven useful in some patients with retinitis and colitis. This drug has many serious side effects, including bone marrow suppression.

Mycobacterioses

The mycobacteriae that are responsible for classic tuberculosis and atypical tuberculosis are appearing with unusual frequency in patients with HIV infection. In these individuals the disease may affect organs other than the lungs and lymph nodes, the general sites of infection in classic tuberculosis. The disease responds in varying degrees to antitubercular agents; drug dosages are generally increased and treatment times extended for patients with HIV.

Another mycobacterium, avium intracellulare, which generally affects birds, commonly infects patients with AIDS. Many parts of the body may be involved, including the lungs, lymph nodes, spleen, bone marrow, and gastrointestinal tract. There is currently no effective treatment for this disease.

Kaposi's Sarcoma (KS)

KS is a formerly rare malignant tumor that can kill directly by attacking vital organs: the lymphatic system, lungs, brain. However, people with AIDS most often succumb to other opportunistic infections. KS in the walls of blood vessels causes dark blue or purple blotches and bumps on the skin, most frequently on the legs and arms, but sometimes also on the chest, back, and face. Lesions are painless until they become large and block circulation. Since this cancer involves the entire body, chemotherapy and radiation cannot cure it. These therapies have, however, been used to slow disease progression.

Pneumocystis carinii Pneumonia

Caused by a parasite, or possibly by a fungus (Altman, 1988), this pneumonia affects the lungs of persons with AIDS and others whose immune systems are not functioning adequately. Its symptoms are those of other types of pneumonia: cough (usually nonproductive), chills, fever, and shortness of breath. Diagnosis is made through a bronchoscopic examination. The disease is associated with high fatality rates among AIDS patients, although treatment success is improving with the development of a variety of new drugs and of improved drug administration methods. At present the drug of choice is pentamidine isethionate.

Toxoplasmosis

Toxoplasmosis is caused by a protozoan that affects the central nervous system. Drugs used to treat this disease at present have serious side effects, and discontinuance frequently leads to reinfection.

Cryptococcosis

Cryptococcosis is caused by a fungus. The disease most frequently causes meningitis, but involvement of the lungs and other organs has been seen. Treatment of choice is presently amphotericin B, administered intravenously. The drug has serious and debilitating side effects and is difficult to deliver intravenously in the arms or legs.

Cryptosporidiosis

Caused by a protozoan, cryptosporidiosis in AIDS patients produces severe diarrhea leading to dehydration, malnutrition, and death; respiratory tract infections may also occur. Transmission is from feces to mouth. There is presently no effective treatment, although new drug therapy is being studied. Nursing care of these patients is of primary importance in maintaining skin integrity, nutrition, hydration, and comfort.

Cofactors of HIV Infection

Cofactors of an event are variables that increase its likelihood. Possible cofactors of symptomatic HIV infection presently under investigation are characteristics or behaviors that may work against a healthy immune system, including use of drugs, an abnormality in the immune system, and repeated or current infection with bacteria or other viruses. Attention to cofactors of HIV infection will not prevent AIDS but may limit the damage the virus will do once it enters the body.

Use of Drugs

- Excessive use of alcohol and other mind-altering drugs promotes risky activities that might be avoided in a state of sobriety.
- Drugs such as alcohol, heroin, and cocaine can directly depress the immune system.

Abnormal Immune System

- The possibility of genetic predisposition to acquired immunodeficiency disorders is being investigated.
- Poor general nutrition can weaken the immune response.
- Treatment with antibiotics over long periods of time may weaken the immune response.
- The role of stress in depressing the immune response has been studied by a number of investigators.

Repeated or Current Infection

- An immune system that has been bombarded by diseases of various kinds may be compromised in its ability to fend off HIV.
- Sexually transmitted diseases that leave large open sores in the genital area (syphilis, herpes) may provide ready portals of entry for HIV.
- The presence of other organisms in the body may increase HIV activity.

Antiviral Therapy for HIV Infection

One antiviral drug, azidothymidine (AZT, zidovudine, Retrovir), has recently been developed and is presently in clinical use for patients with AIDS. Although it has serious side effects in some patients, this drug has prolonged the lives of many people with AIDS. There remains a question concerning who will absorb the cost of this expensive drug—the patient, society, or both.

A particularly promising area of investigation is the interruption of the life cycle of the virus through attempting to block the binding of certain viral proteins to a glycoprotein (CD4) found on the surface of T helper cells (Yarchoan, Mitsuya, & Broder, 1988).

Vaccine Development

A great deal of work is being done to develop and test a vaccine that would render the recipient immune to HIV infection. However, significant problems have been encountered because of the nature of HIV, the ability of the virus to mutate, and its ability to hide in a cell without betraying its presence. Even when trial vaccines are ready to be tested in humans, it is likely that few people will be willing or appropriate subjects for such studies (Matthews & Bolognesi, 1988).

TRANSMISSION

The major routes for transmission of HIV are: (1) sexual, (2) parenteral, and (3) transplacental. Parenteral infection generally refers to transmission through intact skin into the bloodstream, usually by skin prick or needle. This route is also referred to as *percutaneous*. Sexual and parenteral routes of transmission have accounted for the great majority of diagnosed cases of AIDS in the United States. While small amounts of the virus have been found in body fluids such as tears, saliva, urine, and the liquid portion of stool, these fluids have not been implicated in the transmission of HIV.

Since the virus is present in monocytes and T lymphocytes, it is present in all body fluids. However, it is *transmitted* only through sexual contact with an infected person, by sharing needles with an infected person, by transfusion or infusion with infected blood, by an infected mother to a fetus during pregnancy or at birth, or, rarely, by an infected mother to her nursing infant. The virus is not found in sperm but is found in semen, also called seminal fluid, which contains not only sperm but many monocytes.

Pathogens of all kinds are generally transmitted to

humans in one, or occasionally more than one, of the following ways:

- Through sexual contact with an infected person
- Through the respiratory system by breathing organisms from the air
- Through the digestive system by ingesting the organisms
- Through the blood from open skin or mucous membrane exposure, or injection of infected blood

Most pathogens do not have access to all routes of entry. In the case of HIV, the identified routes are through sexual contact and through blood.

To be absolutely certain you do not catch the virus, avoid all forms of sexual contact with infected persons and protect yourself from internal contamination with their blood.

Sexual Transmission

Certain sexual practices carry a high risk of transmitting the virus if one of the partners is infected with it. Other practices carry slight risk.

Behaviors That Can
Transmit the HIV Virus

- Rectal intercourse, especially if preceded by fisting (inserting a hand or fist into the rectum)
- Sharing needles for intravenous injections
- Vaginal intercourse
- Oral sex
- Deep kissing
- Rimming (anal to mouth contact)
- Sharing dildos or other objects that are inserted into body openings
- Douching or using enemas before or after sex, which can weaken the body's natural defenses against infection

Behaviors That Do Not
Transmit Disease

- Talking sexy
- Touching (with no exchange of semen, vaginal fluid, or blood). Gloves may be used. Types of touch may include:

Hugging
Stroking
Cuddling
Caressing
Massaging
Wrestling
Masturbation
Kissing (dry)

Blood Transmission:
Other Than Sexual Activity

The three primary nonsexual means by which HIV directly infects blood in the United States are through blood transfusion or infusion of blood products (before March 1985), through infected needles, and from mother to fetus.

Blood Transfusion

Blood transfusions have not been a major source of infection since March 1985, when the HIV antibody test began to be used on blood donations. The present risk of becoming infected with HIV through a blood transfusion is minimal. When blood is needed in an emergency, the risk of harm to the patient by denying it is far greater than the risk of HIV infection from transfusing donated blood. In many areas blood-collection agencies store autologous (one's own) blood for use in elective surgery. There is no risk to the blood donor of infection with the virus from *giving* blood to a reputable blood bank.

Infected Needles

In some areas of the country the use of infected needles to inject illicit drugs is the most frequent avenue of infection. The most effective way for drug users to protect themselves from AIDS is to end their drug habit. However, professional help and community support will be needed in this effort.

While waiting for acceptance into a drug treatment program, users must be taught how to clean drug paraphernalia ("works"). The program in New York City that provides drug users with clean needles deserves emulation in other metropolitan centers.

Mother to Fetus

The Centers for Disease Control has suggested that all women of childbearing age with identifiable risk of HIV infection should be routinely counseled and tested for HIV antibody. The object of testing would be to encourage the woman to avoid pregnancy if she is HIV positive. Thirty to fifty percent of infants born to HIV-infected women are infected with the virus (Centers for Disease Control, August 14, 1987).

Women at high risk of infection include those who have used IV drugs, have engaged in prostitution, have had sexual partners who are infected or at risk of infection, live or have lived in communities with a high prevalence of infection among women, or have received a blood transfusion in the United States between 1978 and 1985. Counseling preceding such testing should include a clear statement of the risks and benefits of the test to the woman and her family, including potential children. Such counseling is the only way to assure that consent for testing is truly voluntary.

Through voluntary education and testing programs, women who have HIV and are already pregnant will be able to receive appropriate medical care and to plan medical care for their infants. Counseling on family planning, future pregnancies, and the risk of transmitting HIV to others can also be provided.

PREVENTION

Sexual abstinence or a long-standing sexual relationship that is mutually monogamous are protections that uninfected people can use against HIV and other sexually transmitted infections. Sexual intercourse—vaginal, rectal, or oral—with an infected person is dangerous.

Since it is very difficult to know whether another person has HIV infection, protection with a latex condom, latex or well-fitting rubber gloves, or latex oral dam is a good idea. If no other protection is available, flexible plastic food wrap may be used. Use of a spermicidal jelly containing nonoxynol-9 for vaginal or rectal sex may also help to kill the virus. Needles used to inject drugs should never be shared.

Condom Use

Condoms can break, particularly during rectal sex, which is frequently more traumatic to the mucous membranes than is vaginal intercourse. The effectiveness of a condom in preventing disease depends on how it is used.

Choosing and Caring for a Condom

- Use latex condoms only. So-called natural membrane condoms are not effective against viral infection.
- Condoms should be stored in a cool, dry place out of direct sunlight.
- Use only condoms that show no sign of damage. A damaged condom may be brittle or discolored.

Putting on the Condom

- Wash genital area with soap and water.
- Put on condom before any genital contact.
- Place a drop of spermicidal jelly, cream, or foam inside the rolled condom. Do not get lubricant on the shaft of the penis.
- Hold the tip of the condom and unroll it onto the erect penis.
- Leave a space at the tip for collection of semen.
- Be careful not to puncture the condom with fingernails.
- Assure that no air is trapped in the tip of the condom.
- Wear two condoms whenever possible.

Lubricating the Condom

- Use water-based lubricants such as KY jelly. Petroleum-based or oil-based lubricants such as Vaseline, cooking oil, hair grease, shortening, and lotions may weaken the latex and cause failure of the condom.

- Lubrication with a spermicidal jelly containing nonoxynol-9 may provide some added protection.
- Use a small amount of lubricant inside and more lubricant outside the condom.

During and after Intercourse

- Withdrawal before climax is the safest practice.
- If a condom breaks during intercourse, withdraw immediately and put on a new condom before continuing sexual activity.
- After ejaculation, take care that the condom does not slip off the penis before withdrawal. To do this, hold the condom firmly and withdraw while the penis is still erect.
- Remove the condom carefully, well away from partner's genital area.
- Discard immediately in a plastic-lined garbage can or bag.
- Do not reuse condom.
- Wash hands with soap and water after discarding condom.

Cleaning Needles

Intravenous drug users should never use a needle that someone else has used. The following guidelines may be followed.

- Don't go to shooting galleries.
- Don't rent works.
- Use your own clean equipment, and don't let anyone else use it.
- Some needles sold on the street may be packaged as "new" but are actually dirty needles that have been rebagged.
- Needles may be cleaned in the following manner:
    Works should be cleaned immediately before use, even if they were cleaned previously.
    Attach the needle to the syringe.
    Place some full-strength bleach in a cup.
    Draw up a full syringe of bleach, then squirt this into a sink, commode, or garbage can. Repeat one time.

Place some water in a cup.

Draw up a full syringe of water, then squirt this into a sink, commode, or garbage can. Repeat one time.

Do not inject bleach.

BIBLIOGRAPHY

Altman, L. K. (August 14, 1988). New studies point to fungus as leading to AIDS deaths. *New York Times.*

Altman, L. K. (February 5, 1989). Who's stricken and how: AIDS pattern is shifting. *New York Times.*

Brandt, A. M. (1987). A historical perspective. In H. L. Dalton and S. Burris (eds.), *AIDS and the Law,* p. 41. New Haven: Yale University Press.

Centers for Disease Control. AIDS Weekly Surveillance Report. Washington, DC: U.S. Department of Health and Human Services.

Centers for Disease Control (August 14, 1987). Public health service guidelines for counseling and antibody testing to prevent HIV infection and AIDS. *Morbidity and Mortality Weekly Report*: 509–515.

Lewis, A. (1988). Nursing Care of the Person with AIDS/ARC. Rockville, MD: Aspen.

Matthews, T. J., & D. P. Bolognesi (1988). AIDS vaccines. *Scientific American, 259*(4):120–127.

Rowe, M., & C. Ryan (1987). AIDS: A Public Health Challenge, Vol. 3, p. 19. Washington, DC: U.S. Department of Health and Human Services.

Sedaka, S. D., & M. O'Reilly (1986). The financial implications of AIDS. *Caring, V*(6):38–46.

Yarchoan, R., H. Mitsuya, & S. Broder (1988). AIDS therapies. *Scientific American, 259*(4):110–119.

2

PROTECTING YOURSELF AND YOUR PATIENTS

Health care providers and their patients want to be very sure that no transmissible disease is passed between them. This chapter presents information about what health care providers should do to protect themselves and their patients from HIV infection.

Many health care practices have been defined by habit and precedent. These practices have been based on a set of assumptions, one of which is that blood is not likely to be infectious. Today, we can no longer make that assumption. If proper precautions are followed, however, the incidence of transmitting HIV and other blood-borne diseases in a health care situation will be slight.

Since 1981, when AIDS first came to the attention of the Centers for Disease Control (CDC), very few health care workers have tested positive for HIV antibody even after direct exposure to the blood of a patient infected with HIV. Recent information places the risk at only 0.4 percent, or 4 in 1,000, that an HIV-negative health care provider with no risk factors for HIV will convert to HIV positive after a needle-stick injury or a cut with known exposure to HIV-positive blood (Henderson, 1988). Several workers who contracted the virus said they knew what to do to prevent infection, but for one reason or another, failed to take those simple precautions.

Although the health care provider is at greater risk of contracting blood-borne infection than is the average person, experience over the course of the AIDS epidemic has shown that almost all exposures to these infections are preventable. The person with a healthy immune system is also not likely to contract any of the opportunistic diseases that infect AIDS patients.

Many of the daily activities performed by health care providers expose them to some risk of HIV infection. Just as fastening a seatbelt decreases the risk of serious injury in an automobile accident, following certain simple precautions will dramatically lower the risk of contracting an infectious blood-borne disease.

Despite widespread recognition of the value of seatbelts, many drivers and passengers do not buckle up. Similarly, a vaccine to prevent hepatitis B is recommended for all health care providers who come in contact with blood, yet many who give direct patient care have not been vaccinated. Health care providers risk their own health and that of their patients when they don't wash their hands between patients. Nevertheless, sometimes even this simple precaution is ignored.

As you study the guidelines developed to protect you and your patients, remember that if they are to be effective they must be followed consistently. The most important precautions in preventing HIV infection involve handwashing and avoiding injury with needles or other sharp implements that have been contaminated with blood.

GENERAL RISK REDUCTION

The health care provider must act as if the blood of every person is infected and therefore infectious. Do not attempt to be especially careful with patients known to be HIV positive. Since you often will not know who is infected and who is not, such an attitude could lead to taking unreasonable risks.

Since medical history and examination cannot reliably identify all patients infected with blood-borne pathogens, a set of precautions has been suggested by the Centers for Disease Control (CDC) to be used consistently with all patients. This approach, referred to by the CDC as "universal precautions," is intended to prevent percutaneous and mucous membrane exposures of health care workers to blood-borne pathogens. The American Hospital Association supports the use of these universal precautions in all hospitals and health care settings (AHA, 1987–88).

The general guidelines that follow were developed from the August 21, 1987, CDC document, *Recommendations for Prevention of HIV Transmission in Health-Care Settings,* and the supplementary guidelines, U.S. Public Health Service, *Morbidity and Mortality Weekly Report,* June 24, 1988, Vol. 37, No. 24. Two other useful resources for specific circumstances are *Nursing Care of the Person with AIDS/ARC* (Lewis, 1988) and *AIDS* (De Vita *et al.,* 1988), listed in the reference section at the end of this chapter.

Certain body fluids are not considered infectious for blood-borne disease unless they contain visible blood. These include feces, nasal secretions, sputum, sweat, tears, urine, and vomitus. Health care providers in contact with any of these body substances may, of course, wear gloves for esthetic reasons or to prevent transfer of infectious organisms transmitted by routes other than blood.

In the following discussion, the term "gloves" means intact latex or vinyl gloves, either sterile or nonsterile as the situation dictates. The term "gowns" means gowns that are impervious to liquids. The Occupational Safety and Health Administration has provided standards for gloves and other barrier apparel and equipment (OSHA, August 1988).

Handwashing

- Wash hands immediately and thoroughly before performing invasive procedures or if they come in contact with blood or bloody secretions or with linens, dressings, or trash soiled with blood. Use a mild soap and water followed by lotion to help prevent drying and cracking of your skin.
- For performing procedures under special circumstances, such as before surgery or in newborn nurseries or intensive care units, use the special handwashing agent and procedure identified by your agency policy.

Gloves

- Wear gloves for touching blood, nonintact mucous membrane, broken skin, bloody linens or dressings, and trash contaminated with blood. Wash your hands immediately before putting on gloves and discard gloves after use in appropriate containers at the patient's bedside. Wash your hands immediately after removing gloves.

- Change gloves between patients.
- If gloves are punctured or torn in use, remove as quickly as possible within the patient situation, wash your hands, and put on a new pair of gloves.
- Double-gloving is usually not necessary; it would not prevent punctures or cuts.

Masks and Protective Eyewear

- Wear masks and protective eyewear (goggles or glasses) or face shields to prevent exposure of mucous membranes of the mouth, nose, and eyes during procedures in which blood may spatter.
- Wear masks and protective eyewear or face shields when caring for a patient who is producing sputum with visible blood or who needs any type of suctioning likely to produce bleeding.
- Wear both masks and eyewear; neither offers sufficient protection alone.
- If you wear glasses, special goggles are generally not necessary. Spattered personal eyeglasses may be cleaned with soap and water and germicide.

Gowns or Aprons

- Wear a waterproof gown or apron during procedures in which clothing is likely to be contaminated with blood. A waterproof apron may be worn under water-permeable sterile attire.
- If gowns are soiled with blood they should be changed as soon as reasonable within the patient care situation.
- Discard disposable gowns in the plastic-lined container near the patient's bedside.

Handling Laboratory Specimens

- All laboratory specimens should be transported in well-constructed containers with secure lids to prevent leaking.
- Handle laboratory specimens with gloves and label them

according to your agency policy. Be sure that the outside of the specimen container and the laboratory form accompanying the specimen are kept clean.

- Transport specimen containers in plastic bags with secure closures to prevent leakage or breakage if the container should be dropped. The laboratory request form should be attached to the outside of the plastic bag.

Handling Soiled Linens

- Place linens in leak-proof bags at the bedside. They should not be sorted or rinsed in patient care areas.
- Soiled linens should be transported in bags that prevent leakage.
- Handling of linens in hospitals or other health care agencies should follow institutional, local, and state guidelines.
- If hot water is used, linen should be washed with detergent in water at least 71°C (160°F) for 25 minutes. If low-temperature laundry cycles are used, proper concentrations of chemicals suitable for low-temperature washing should be used.

Needles and Sharp Instruments

- Needles, sharp instruments, syringes and intravenous equipment with needles attached, and any tube that has been soiled with blood should be handled with extraordinary care.
- Never manipulate used needles by hand. This means:
    Do not recap needles.
    Do not purposely bend or break needles.
    Do not remove needles from disposable syringes.
- Place used disposable syringes and needles, scalpel blades, and other sharp items in puncture-resistant containers, which should be kept as close as possible to places where these instruments are used. Cardboard boxes should not be used to dispose of needles and sharp items. Containers should be located at or below eye level for good visibility and should be emptied when they are two-thirds to three-fourths full.

- Needles and sharp items should be disposed of by the person using them.
- Large-bore reusable needles should be placed in a puncture-resistant container for transport to a reprocessing area.
- Only needle-locking syringes or one-piece needle-syringe units should be used to aspirate fluids from patients.

Providing Direct Care

- Do not provide direct patient care or handle patient care equipment if you have oozing, open areas on your skin. Fitness for duty is determined by institutional policy. You should consult your health officer or private physician.
- Use gloves for providing personal care that may bring you in contact with body fluids—for example, in washing the genital area or brushing teeth (if bleeding of the gums is possible).
- Use gloves, either sterile or nonsterile, depending on the correct protocol, for procedures in which bleeding is expected. Such procedures include changing or irrigating catheters where fresh blood is present, caring for decubitus or other types of ulcers, changing dressings, starting or discontinuing intravenous fluids, and hanging blood.

Mouth-to-Mouth Resuscitation

- Mouthpieces, resuscitation bags, or other ventilation devices should be available for use in areas in which the need for resuscitation is predictable. These areas include offices, hospital entrances, and patient's rooms. Use these whenever possible in an emergency.
- Keep a disposable mouthpiece ready for use in a plastic bag in the pocket of your uniform.

Pregnant Health Care Providers

- Pregnant health care providers should adhere strictly to the above precautions. There is no evidence that they are at greater risk of contracting HIV infection than nonpregnant providers.

- Cytomegalovirus, a pathogen common in patients with depressed immune systems, is dangerous to a fetus. However, this virus is transmitted in the same manner as HIV, so that the usual precautions protect against it. Pregnant women are nonetheless advised not to provide direct care to patients who are actively shedding CMV.

Spills

- Visible material should be removed with gloved hands and paper towels, and the area cleaned with soap and water.
- Areas contaminated with large amounts of blood and porous surfaces should be cleaned with a fresh (prepared daily) solution of 1:10 household bleach and water or other germ-killing solution provided by the agency or hospital. A weaker bleach solution may be used for general cleaning of nonporous areas contaminated with small amounts of blood. For this purpose, a dilution of 1:100 should suffice (Henderson, 1988). This dilution may be obtained by adding 2 teaspoons of bleach to 1 quart of water.
- Be very careful when mixing concentrated bleach with water. Refrain from breathing the fumes by holding your face well back from the mixing area. Breathing concentrated chlorine bleach fumes can result in swelling of the throat and in other harmful reactions.
- In mixing bleach and water, put the water in the container first, then the bleach.
- Be very careful in any patient care setting not to mix chlorine bleach with ammonia. Toxic fumes can be generated if, for instance, bleach solution and an ammonia-containing toilet bowl cleaner are mixed when the bleach solution is flushed down a commode. Breathing these fumes could result in serious damage to the lungs, liver, or blood-producing organs.
- Caution patients and families about mixing ammonia-containing cleaners and bleach water in drains, sinks, commodes, or tubs.

Managing Exposures to Blood

- Information about protocols to use when a health care provider has sustained a needle-stick injury or other work-related exposure to blood may be obtained by calling the CDC Hospital Infections Program at (404) 639-1644.
- If a health care provider is exposed percutaneously (through the skin) or through the mucous membrane (by a splash to the eye or mouth) to blood or has had skin exposure involving large amounts of blood or prolonged contact with blood, your agency protocol should be followed. The patient should be informed of the incident and, after informed consent is obtained, should be tested for serologic evidence of HIV infection. Policies of the agency should be followed related to testing of patients in situations in which consent cannot be obtained (for example, an unconscious patient) or when the patient refuses testing.
- If the source patient has AIDS, is positive for HIV antibody, or refuses the test, the health care provider who has been exposed should be counseled by a physician regarding the risk of infection and should be evaluated for evidence of HIV infection as soon as possible after the exposure. Testing soon after exposure will establish the current HIV status of the health care provider. Later testing, on a schedule set by the agency, would be needed to discover a change in antibody status from negative to positive, an indication of HIV infection. The usual testing schedule is 6 weeks, 3 months, 6 months, and 12 months after exposure (Henderson, 1988).
- The exposed health care provider should seek medical evaluation for any acute illness with fever that occurs within 12 weeks after the exposure. An illness characterized by fever, rash, or enlarged lymph nodes may indicate recent HIV infection. The provider should also practice behaviors that will protect sexual partners.
- Further follow-up should follow the protocol outlined by the CDC in the August 21, 1987, guidelines and supplementary recommendations and should be done under the direction of a physician.

- Health care providers should remember that prolonged exposure of a patient to the blood of an infected health care provider could transmit the virus to the patient. Although such exposure is extremely unlikely, if it occurs the patient may request that the health care provider be tested for HIV antibody.

Assessment of Vital Signs

In addition to the above guidelines, which are based on directives from the Centers for Disease Control, certain precautions should be taken when assessing a patient's vital signs. The following precautions reflect good general practice and common sense.

- If blood pressure cuffs become contaminated with blood, the outer cuff should be removed and washed. The bladder should be cleaned with alcohol or as directed by the manufacturer. There should be extra covers for blood pressure cuffs on each patient care unit.
- The head of the stethoscope should be cleaned with alcohol between patients.
- Patients should have personal thermometers and these should be used whenever possible; otherwise, a thermometer with a disposable cover should be used.

RISK REDUCTION
IN SPECIAL SETTINGS

Beyond the general precautions detailed above, certain additional precautions should be taken in specialty areas.

General Medical-Surgical Units

Patients on general medical-surgical units in hospitals often receive fluids and medications through a variety of tubes. Sometimes these patients become confused and pull out their tubing, causing bleeding. Gloves should be used when handling the tubing attached to agitated patients.

Health care providers working with patients with gastrointestinal bleeding are frequently concerned about the possibility of infection from blood in vomitus or fecal material. HIV-positive blood that has gone through the digestive process is not infectious. However, infection might be transmitted by fresh blood coming from the mouth or esophagus. All vomitus, sputum, saliva, feces, and urine containing visible blood must be considered potentially dangerous and handled with gloves.

Patients who have had nasogastric tubes in place for long periods of time may bleed through the nose and may require nasal packing to stop the bleeding. Soiled nasal packing must be considered infectious.

Patients with central lines and multiple venous and arterial access ports present many opportunities for health care providers to come in contact with blood. Consistent use of gloves will prevent infection in these situations.

Transporting a patient who is walking, in a wheelchair, or on a wheeled bed should not be a problem. No patient needs to wear special attire unless he has, or is believed to have, an infection that is transmitted through the air, such as active pulmonary tuberculosis.

Recapping a needle or carrying an uncapped needle and syringe outside a patient's room for disposal should never be necessary. Some container to hold used needles must be available in each room, or the needles must be inserted into a protective device such as a piece of foam in order to transport them. Containers for needle disposal must be emptied before they are full.

Operating Room

Hospitals generally provide guidelines for preventing transmission of blood-borne infections in the operating room. These should be consistent with current CDC guidelines.

The CDC has identified the following fluids as coming under the same guidelines for universal precautions as blood: cerebrospinal fluid, synovial fluid, pleural fluid, peritoneal fluid, pericardial fluid, and amniotic fluid.

Operating room staff should follow agency guidelines when invasive procedures are called for. The CDC guidelines (August 1987) define an invasive procedure as:

surgical entry into the tissues, cavities or organs or 1) repair of major traumatic injuries in an operating or delivery room, emergency department, or outpatient setting, including both physicians' and dentists' offices; 2) cardiac catheterization and angiographic procedures; 3) a vaginal or caesarean delivery or other invasive obstetric procedure during which bleeding may occur; or 4) the manipulation, cutting, or removal of any oral or perioral tissues, including tooth structure, during which bleeding occurs or the potential for bleeding exists (Centers for Disease Control, August 21, 1987).

Specific guidelines for health care providers in the operating room generally include:

- Routinely use barrier precautions to prevent skin and mucous membrane contact with blood and other body fluids identified above.
- Use gloves for all invasive procedures.
- Use masks and protective eyewear for any procedure in which blood is likely to spatter.
- If a glove is torn or a needlestick or other injury to the hand occurs, gloves should be removed, hands washed, and new gloves put on as promptly as patient safety permits.
- Soiled needles or other instruments should not be allowed to contaminate the sterile field.
- Invasive patient care equipment should be disposable or should be sterilized. Such equipment includes laryngoscopes, bronchoscopes, endoscopes, endotracheal tubes, and other instruments that come in contact with blood, secretions, excretions, or tissues. These should be sterilized by steam under pressure before reuse. The list also includes lensed instruments, which should be sterilized by ethylene oxide or activated glutaraldehyde before reuse.
- Health care providers with extensive dermatitis should not provide direct patient care.

Dialysis

In addition to general precautions, health care providers working in renal dialysis units should follow the guidelines set forth in the *Morbidity and Mortality Weekly Report*, August 21, 1987.

- Universal precautions should be used by all staff members for all activities involved in dialyzing *all* patients.
- There is no need to isolate HIV-positive patients who are being dialyzed by either hemodialysis or peritoneal dialysis.
- Strategies already accepted for cleaning the fluid pathways of dialyzing machines are sufficient.
- Centers that reuse dialyzers on the same patient, after disinfection, may include HIV-infected patients in this program.
- An individual dialyzer must never be used on more than one patient.
- Masks, goggles, gowns, and gloves should be worn when attaching and removing dialyzing equipment, including continuous ambulatory peritoneal dialysis (CAPD) equipment.

Labor and Delivery

In the labor and delivery suites, the same precautions should be followed as in the operating room. In addition, the following special guidelines should be used.

Protective Gear and Equipment

- Wear gown, gloves, or both when:
  Handling a placenta or touching amniotic fluid
  Handling the infant until the blood and amniotic fluid have been removed from the baby's skin
  Drawing or running cord blood gases
  Weighing or handling the placenta or cord
  Handling the baby prior to its first bath
  Changing bloody or soiled dressings and linens
  Coming in contact with wound drainage
- Protective clothing that is contaminated with blood should be changed as soon as possible.
- Masks and protective eyewear should be worn for:
  Rupturing membranes
  Drawing cord blood gases

Postpartum Unit

In the postpartum unit, handwashing is the strategy that is likely to be most effective in preventing transmission of disease. Hands should be washed after changing protective bed pads, sanitary napkins, or bloody linens, and after any skin contact with blood or other body fluids that have been identified as dangerous.

Newborn Nursery

Since handwashing and gloving are procedures in general use in infant nurseries, general and special precautions for labor and delivery should serve to prevent blood-borne infection.

It should be noted that while infected breast milk has been implicated in the transmission of HIV from mother to infant, breast milk, unless it contains visible blood, is not considered infectious to the health care provider.

Emergency Medical Services (EMS)

Persons working on emergency medical teams or on mobile trauma units frequently encounter bleeding patients. Sharp objects such as pieces of metal or splinters of wood are often present at the scene of an accident. Workers should take special precautions not to injure themselves.

Many people who need the help of the EMS worker require resuscitation, which could permit the transfer of blood by mouth. The following guidelines should be used in emergency situations.

Protective Gear

- Disposable mouthpieces (units) for resuscitation should be used in every instance. These should be carried by all health care providers in a plastic bag in a pocket.
- Disposable resuscitation bags and intubation equipment should be used whenever possible.

- Emergency workers must assume that every call will require protective garb—gloves, waterproof apron, mask, and goggles. These should be used in any situation where blood is likely to spatter.
- Laypersons assisting in an emergency should be provided with appropriate gear (usually gloves) for the task. Volunteers are often called upon, for example, to hold a pressure dressing on a bleeding wound.

*Cleaning and Disposing
of Equipment*

- The equipment in the emergency care vehicle should be cleaned thoroughly after each patient with a fresh solution of bleach and water or with hospital-approved disinfectant. Gloves and paper towels should be used for this purpose and should be discarded afterward in plastic bags.
- Care must be taken to dispose of needles and other sharp instruments. Needles should not be recapped.
- Commercial portable containers are available to dispose of used needles at the scene of an accident, but an empty bleach bottle can serve quite well as a portable disposal unit.
- It is important not to leave bloody dressings at the scene. Gross blood on objects should be wiped up, unless police rule otherwise.

Hospice and Home Care

Hospice and home health care providers need to take certain special precautions against transmission of blood-borne infections. These are listed below.

Cleaning

- When the home has no running water for handwashing, take a jug of clean water with you.
- Keep a bottle of fresh bleach and water solution with you. Any patient who is likely to have spills of blood should also have his own fresh solution at home.

Protective Gear and Equipment

- Use gloves to draw blood, to start and stop intravenous infusions, and to hang blood.
- Keep gloves, moisture-proof gowns, masks, goggles, and disposable resuscitation mouth shields available with the equipment you carry.

Disposing of Needles and Used Equipment

- Dispose of needles in a container that you carry into the home with you. It is not acceptable to leave used needles in the patient's home.
- Needles the patient uses on himself may be safely placed into a bleach bottle or coffee can with a lid and discarded when the container is full in the patient's plastic or metal garbage container.
- If a coffee can is used, the container may be taped before disposal, or it may be baked for 30 minutes in a 400-degree oven (to melt the syringes and prevent reuse), or it may be taken to a central location for disposal (Dickinson et al., 1988, p. 221). State and local guidelines are being developed for residents of specific communities.
- Under no circumstances should used needles and syringes be transported in the nurse's duty bag.
- Carry extra plastic bags for disposal of soiled disposable bed pads, dressings, urine containers, catheters, colostomy drainage bags, oxygen tubing, and suction tubing. This bag should be placed in another bag in a collection container with a tight lid in the patient's home.

Disposing of Wastes

- Tissues, soiled dressings, used tampons and sanitary pads, and diapers should be discarded in a plastic-lined wastebasket. The plastic bag should then be placed in a garbage bag and then in a garbage can with a tight-fitting lid.
- Blood and body wastes can be poured down the drain connected to a sanitary sewage system. In rural areas without such systems, consult the local health department for advice.

- Take special care in disposing of the contents of containers used to collect sputum after suctioning if the sputum contains blood. Sputum may be carefully poured into the toilet bowl.

Taking Vital Signs

- Each patient should have a personal thermometer, which should be washed with soap and water after each use.
- Keep extra outer cuffs available to use if a blood pressure cuff becomes soiled with blood.

Giving Personal Care

- Only electric or disposable razors should be used in patient care.
- Use gloves for any care that involves touching blood, vaginal fluid, or secretions containing blood.

Emergency Guidelines for Accidental
Ingestion of Bleach Solution

- Emergency care guidelines for accidental ingestion of bleach solution should be provided to each patient. These guidelines are presented below.

Nursing Homes

Health care providers in nursing homes and some employers have tended to dismiss HIV infection as something that does not affect nursing home patients. However, before March 1985, when the American Red Cross began to test blood for HIV antibody, some older people received contaminated blood. Some older people have been sexually active or used IV drugs within the past ten years and have been infected with HIV. These people are now beginning to have symptoms of immune suppression.

Patient care providers in nursing homes should follow the same guidelines as providers in hospitals. Gloves, masks, gowns, aprons, and disposable mouth protectors should be used as with any other patient in the hospital or the home. Needles and sharp items should be disposed of in accordance with CDC guidelines.

Psychiatric Inpatient Facilities

In most cases psychiatric patients do not present any greater risk to health care providers or to each other than does any other group of patients. However, a growing number of HIV-positive persons are showing signs of impaired judgment and unpredictable behavior.

An often-stated concern of staff is that a patient may bite someone (the staff or another patient). This rarely happens. If it does, remember that for the virus to be transmitted there would have to be cuts or tears in the lining of the biter's mouth, and the biter's blood would have to commingle in the wound with the wounded person's blood. If bitten, a health care provider should always follow the first-aid guidelines of the American Red Cross:

- Milk the wound to make it bleed.
- Wash well with soap and water.
- Seek the advice of a medical professional.

Health care providers cannot overlook the possibility of sexual activity between patients. Many psychiatric patients would not be likely to use condoms even if they were provided. And although IV drug use does not occur on most psychiatric units, where it does, patients are more likely than other users to share needles. It is necessary to be vigilant in supervising patients at all times of the day and night.

The health care provider has to believe in the possibility that high-risk activities may occur and that patients are telling the truth if they say that these things have happened. There are obvious legal risks if the health care provider ignores such information and a patient is subsequently harmed.

Confidentiality related to diagnosis of HIV status takes on special aspects in a psychiatric unit. A physician may decide to give information about the HIV status of patients who cannot control their behavior to staff

(including nonprofessional staff) and to community
workers when the patient is discharged. The responsibility for this decision rests with the primary care provider.

These sensitive issues are appropriate subjects for discussion in group sessions by all concerned, including patient groups. Records of discussions by staff and patients,
along with any education that is provided, should be kept
by the organization. Health care providers should initiate
discussions with administrators in their organizations so
that practical policy decisions may be made.

Preschool Day Care Settings

While the political and social battles rage on about
whether or not children who are known to be HIV positive
should be in school, the fact is that transmission from one
child to another is extremely unlikely. We will address here
the issue of dealing with preschoolers who are HIV positive but not sick, at least not so sick that they can't be
around other children.

Even though an infected person has the virus in all body
fluids (vomitus, sweat, tears, saliva, urine, and feces), no
one has been known to become HIV positive from exposure to a body fluid other than blood, semen, or vaginal
fluid. Good sanitation practices make it necessary to clean
surfaces of any body fluids and excrement. These precautions are taken not primarily because of HIV infection but
because of the possibility of transmitting the many other
diseases that can infect small children in day care settings.

In addition to frequent and careful handwashing, the
following precautions should be followed when providing
health care in day care situations.

Cleaning Spills

- Preschool health care providers should keep a fresh solution (1:10) of chlorine bleach and water on hand to wipe
  up spills. Weaker solutions, as mentioned earlier, are appropriate to wipe up small spills on nonporous surfaces.
- The strength of the solution should be clearly marked on
  the containers.

- Keep the solution well away from the children.
- Use paper towels to wipe up spills.

Accidental Ingestion of
Bleach Solution

- Do not induce vomiting.
- Administer milk or water to dilute the solution and to coat the esophagus.
- Try to prevent coughing in order to avoid aspiration of the chemical.
- Notify the local poison control center immediately, and report the amount and strength of the ingested solution. The center will advise on further treatment.

Disposal of Soiled Diapers

- Dispose of diapers and soiled bandages in a plastic bag placed in a large garbage bag.

First Aid

- Wash small cuts and scratches with soap and water and apply a small bandage.
- Gloves should be readily available to use in managing serious accidents involving blood.

Excluding Children or Teachers from School

- Children with eczema or large areas of weeping skin should be evaluated by a physician for a decision on school attendance.
- Teachers and other health care providers with eczema or large areas of weeping skin should not provide direct care to children until the condition has cleared.

Primary and Secondary Schools

While there is no universal right to education in the United States, there is a right to equal *opportunity* for education. Since, under most circumstances, HIV infection of a classmate poses no danger to uninfected children and teachers, increasing numbers of children and teachers within the school system will be HIV positive. Civil cases that have been brought before the courts have supported the position that, except in the rare case of a hyperaggressive child, HIV-positive primary and secondary school children should not be segregated from their classmates.

Health care providers within the primary and secondary school systems should adhere to general guidelines and should pay particular attention to the following measures.

Equipment

- Assure that all teachers and classroom and playground assistants carry gloves to manage profuse bleeding after accidental injury.
- Assure that all teachers and classroom and playground assistants carry a mouth shield to use in giving mouth-to-mouth resuscitation to an injured student who is bleeding from the mouth, or where resuscitation efforts might result in bleeding.
- Assure that closed units for disposal of sanitary napkins are available in women's restrooms and that these units are emptied and cleaned regularly.

Emergency Equipment

- Disposable mouthpieces and bags used to deliver oxygen in a situation of cardiac arrest should be immediately available.
- Directions for treatment of accidental ingestion of bleach solution should be posted in appropriate places in the school.

Cleaning

- Fresh solutions of bleach solution should be available and clearly labeled.
- Appropriate precautions should be followed in preparing and storing bleach and water solutions.

Patient Care

- Use electronic thermometers with covers or glass thermometers with plastic covers. Glass thermometers should be disinfected between uses.
- Wash hands before and after caring for any student.

Emergency Room Care of
Rape Victims and Victims of
Domestic Violence

Victims of rape and domestic violence should be treated like other trauma victims, but with the following special considerations.

Use of Protective Gear

- Use gloves to handle all clothing and towels that are soiled with blood or semen.
- Provide gloves to laypersons who accompany the patient if there is any chance they will touch blood or semen in helping to care for the patient.

Counseling/Testing

The health care provider should find out whether the patient has considered that HIV infection may have been transmitted in the attack. One of the victim's options is to have an HIV test done to determine present antibody status; tests should be repeated 3, 6, and 12 months later. The patient's specific consent should be obtained before an HIV antibody test is done. Victims of violence need to be reminded that:

- They have a right to refuse testing or to go to an anonymous testing center.
- Testing has social, economic, and legal implications. In some states, insurance may be denied if a person was tested for HIV, whether test results were negative or positive.

- The risk of acquiring HIV infection in rape will depend on which sexual acts were forced on the victim. Traumatic rectal penetration with ejaculation, for instance, is a bigger risk than either vaginal or oral penetration.

Shelters for Domestic Violence Victims

Victims of domestic violence residing in shelters are in crisis and need a great deal of support in dealing with daily living. Often health care in shelters is provided by professional social workers and volunteers rather than by persons specifically trained to provide health care.

Women and children in shelters often have recent wounds that have broken the skin. They may also have vaginal or rectal bleeding.

Managing Blood Spills or Bloody Dressings

- Have wound dressings available, along with plastic bags to dispose of soiled dressings.
- Tampons and sanitary napkin disposal units should be available. These should be hung fairly high on walls so that young children can't reach them.
- A fresh (daily) supply of dilute bleach solution should be available to clients and health care providers. The container should be clearly marked and should be kept well away from children.
- Volunteers who provide emergency safe housing for victims of domestic violence should have gloves available and should be instructed in cleansing procedures, including the safe way to mix fresh bleach solution.
- Protocol for treatment of accidental ingestion of bleach solution should be prominently displayed.

Washing Dishes, Linens, and Clothes

- Dishwashing by hand in hot water will kill HIV. Most shelters comply with state and local health laws that govern washing dishes in public places; this generally means that dishwashers are used.

- Bloody linens should be handled with gloves.
- Place linens in bags at the bedside.
- Transport soiled linens in bags that prevent leakage.
- If hot water is used, linens may be washed with detergent at the regular cycle, which usually means at least 71°C (160°F) for 25 minutes.
- If low-temperature laundry cycles are used, chemicals suitable for low-temperature washing should be used in proper concentrations.

Client Records

- No information concerning HIV status or testing should appear in a client's record. General counseling concerning testing should be recorded.

Shelters for Homeless

Care of homeless people commonly involves bathing, washing clothing and linens, cleaning and dressing wounds, taking temperatures with a mercury or electronic thermometer, and taking blood pressures. All precautions used by health care providers in the home and in safe shelters for women and children should be followed. In addition, the following guidelines should prove useful.

Personal Contact

- Gloves should be worn during personal contact with persons who have bleeding.
- A waterproof apron may be necessary when bathing the person or changing dressings.

Cleaning

- A fresh bleach solution should be available.
- Bleach solution and other cleaning supplies should be clearly marked and kept in locked cabinets.

Supervision

- Policies developed for shelters must take into account awareness that sexual activity and sharing of needles for drug injection can go on in shelters.
- Directions for treatment of accidental ingestion of bleach solution should be prominently posted.

Disposal of Used Equipment

- Hypodermic needles used to administer prescribed medication should be disposed of in an impermeable container such as an empty bleach bottle or coffee can with a lid.
- Needle containers should be kept in a locked cabinet or removed from the shelter daily. Disposal may follow recommendations for providing care in patients' homes.

Halfway Houses

Generally, the health care needs of residents of halfway houses for juveniles, prisoners on parole, or developmentally delayed people are provided by the residence worker. These providers should follow general guidelines and the guidelines for shelter residents. Special precautions may be dictated by consideration of the special needs of the population served. A most important aspect of protection of the health of both residents and care providers is easy access to health care information and the advice of a health care professional.

Industrial Settings

Guidelines for emergency medical service providers should be followed in industrial settings. In addition, the following guidelines may apply:

Protective Apparel and Equipment

- Gloves and disposable mouth shields should be readily available to all workers to use in giving first aid in an emergency.

- Disposable resuscitation bags should be available in all work areas.
- Clearly marked fresh bleach solution should be available.

Physicians' Offices

Since health care providers in physicians' offices are often not professional nurses, the physician must supervise the education of the staff. All general guidelines should be followed and the following additional precautions taken:

- Gloves must be used routinely by office staff for changing bloody linens, bagging linens for laundry, disposing of trash, and cleaning commodes and sinks.
- Clearly labeled fresh bleach solution should be available. Appropriate precautions should be used in preparing it.
- Restroom disposal units for soiled tampons and sanitary pads should be well out of reach of children.
- There should be no open wastebaskets in examining rooms.
- After use needles should be placed immediately, uncapped, into a safe disposal unit.
- Disposable mouthpieces and bags used to deliver oxygen in cases of cardiac arrest should be readily available.

Prisons

Corrections officers are frequently in contact with prisoners' spit, feces, urine, and blood. They should pay meticulous attention to the cleanliness measures detailed in this book, including the use of gloves whenever contact with blood is expected and careful handwashing afterward. Transmission of HIV is usually preventable.

Health care providers in prisons have special opportunities to educate about prevention of HIV infection. Understandably, however, prisons present unique challenges to the provider with respect to HIV prevention. Confidentiality is difficult to maintain in prisons, and the lack of it sometimes has painful consequences. Male HIV-positive prisoners are frequently assumed to be homosexual by other prisoners and may be targets for aggressive acts. Those who are HIV negative may be victims of sexual assault because they are "clean."

Because many prisoners are known to have used intravenous drugs and to be sexually active in prison, opportunities to transmit HIV are relatively frequent. Yet condoms, which could be used to prevent HIV and other sexually transmitted diseases, are rarely available.

Though needles are forbidden, prisoners frequently have them and use them to inject illicit drugs and to apply tattoos. Because they are concealed, it is very difficult to monitor their use. Inevitably in such a situation, "outfits" are not sterilized between uses.

Health care providers working in prison systems must behave as if all inmates were HIV positive, sexually active, and using IV drugs. General guidelines for prevention of blood-borne infections should be used.

Employee Health Services

Providers who work in employee health services should follow the general guidelines for protection. Other expectations may be placed upon them by their employer. Providers should be sure they understand their role in counseling, teaching, information gathering, and recording. These responsibilities should be clarified in writing by the employer.

BIBLIOGRAPHY

American Hospital Association (1987–88). AIDS/HIV infection: Recommendations for health care practices and public policy. *AHA Report.* Chicago: American Hospital Association.

Centers for Disease Control (August 21, 1987). Recommendations for prevention of HIV transmission in health-care settings. *Morbidity and Mortality Weekly Report* (suppl. no. 25), pp. 35–125.

Centers for Disease Control (June 24, 1988). Update: Universal precautions. *Morbidity and Mortality Weekly Report,* p. 378.

De Vita, V. T., S. Hellman, & S. A. Rosenberg (eds.) (1988). AIDS, 2nd ed. Philadelphia: J. B. Lippincott.

Dickinson, D., C. M. F. Clark, & M. J. G. Swafford (1988). AIDS nursing care in the home. In A. Lewis (ed.), *Nursing Care of the Person with AIDS/ARC.* Rockville, MD: Aspen.

Henderson, D. K. (September/October 1988). AIDS and the health-care worker: Management of human immunodeficiency virus infection in the health-care setting. *AIDS Updates,* 1:1–12.

Lewis, A. (1988). Nursing Care of the Person with AIDS/ARC. Rockville, MD: Aspen.

Occupational Safety and Health Administration (August 1988). Instruction CPL 2-2.44A: Enforcement procedures for occupational exposure to hepatitis B virus (HBV) and human immunodeficiency virus (HIV). Washington, DC: U.S. Department of Labor.

U.S. Department of Labor, Department of Health and Human Services. Joint advisory notice (October 30, 1987). HBV/HIV. *Federal Register,* 52:41818–41824.

3

THE TEST

This chapter presents information about the test used to identify HIV-positive individuals, its development, its purpose, and its use in different situations. The specificity and sensitivity of tests and seroconversion are discussed in relation to the controversial issues regarding the test. Testing issues confronting society are presented.

DEVELOPMENT OF THE TEST

In the United States the disease now known as AIDS was first recognized in 1981 among gay males who reported having rectal intercourse with several partners. These men also had histories of infection with other sexually transmitted diseases, such as hepatitis B, cytomegalovirus, syphilis, chlamydial infections, gonorrhea, and genital herpes. AIDS was later identified in recipients of blood and blood products, in infants whose mothers were infected, in intravenous drug users, and in sexual partners of HIV-positive people. This epidemiologic history led public health officials to assume that the infectious agent would be found in blood and semen.

In fact, the human immunodeficiency virus (HIV), which causes AIDS, can be isolated in cultures of many cellular and body fluid samples. But the test for HIV that has been developed and extensively studied uses blood and identifies not the virus but antibodies to it. Antibodies to any pathogen are unique and are not present in the blood unless the body has been invaded by the disease-causing organism.

In the United States a series of three tests done on a single sample of blood is the most common means of identifying HIV antibody. An enzyme-linked immunoabsorbent assay (ELISA) is done and, if it produces positive results, is repeated; if the result of the second ELISA is positive, a Western blot test is done. Only when the series of three tests is positive is the person tested considered HIV positive. All HIV-positive blood is presumed to be infected and infectious.

THE ANTIBODY TEST

Before the antibody test became available for use in March of 1985, there was no way to tell whether the blood donated for transfusions carried the virus. It was largely for the purpose of testing donated blood that an assay for HIV antibody was developed.

Specificity and Sensitivity

A good test is highly *specific* and highly *sensitive*. "Specific" means it identifies the element looked for, and "sensitive" means it identifies almost all occurrences of the element.

Hardly any test is 100% specific or 100% sensitive. An HIV test that identifies something other than HIV is falsely positive, and one that misses an occurrence of HIV is falsely negative.

The Series of Tests Presently Used to Identify HIV

The ELISA, presently made by several different companies, is a very sensitive test. That is, it produces very few false-negative results. It therefore offers assurance that HIV-positive blood can be identified and removed from blood banks. The ELISA does, however, produce some false-positive results; that is, it occasionally identifies as HIV something that is not HIV. Because the implications of carrying HIV are exceedingly grave, the set, or series, of tests currently in use was designed to reduce the possibility of false-positive results.

The ELISA test is relatively inexpensive, costing generally between $2 and $10. The confirming Western blot, however, costs considerably more and is difficult and time-consuming to perform. The expense of the series is one reason why public officials have not bent to public pressure to test large numbers of people.

SEROCONVERSION

A *seronegative* state is one in which a person's blood serum shows no evidence of a particular infection, in this case HIV. *Seropositive* blood shows evidence of infection. The process of going from a seronegative state to a seropositive state is called *seroconversion*. During seroconversion, a person's serum converts from being HIV negative to being HIV positive.

Time It Takes to Convert

Although infection probably occurs as soon as the virus enters the body, it takes several weeks or months for serum to show antibody as measured by currently used tests. This process of *seroconversion* usually takes from 6 to 12 weeks (Centers for Disease Control, August 14, 1987) but may take a year or more (Curran *et al.,* 1985). During this period infected people test negative for the virus but are capable of transmitting it.

Some people who might be expected to become infected have not become seropositive even years after exposure. In these people, the virus is either "hiding" (latent) or is truly not present.

The Difference between Seroconversion and Incubation

The period of time between infection and seroconversion should not be confused with the *incubation period* of the disease. The incubation period is the length of time between infection (when the virus first enters the blood) and the time when a diagnosis of an HIV-related condition or of a disease such as AIDS is made. In the case of AIDS, the incubation period is presently considered to be between 2 and 15 years (Mann *et al.,* 1988).

ACCURACY OF THE TEST

In order to be as certain as possible that results are accurate, tests must be conducted in laboratories with proper equipment and controls and by competent laboratory technicians. Some states require special laboratory licensing for HIV testing.

The test has been found to be *very accurate* in screening donated blood, semen, ova, breast milk, and organs. Occasionally, however, an organ must be transplanted before tests can be completed and the physician must make a judgment about the likelihood of HIV infection. Other tests for use in such emergency circumstances are presently being developed.

The test is also very accurate when used in high-risk groups in which many people have the virus. People who have practiced high-risk behaviors can be confident that their test results are accurate.

On the other hand, when the test is used to screen a large group of people at low risk of carrying HIV, a significant number of false-positive results may occur (Dalton *et al.*, 1987). The CDC states, however, that when the testing *sequence* described above is used, the probability of obtaining false-positive results in a population with a low rate of infection is low (Centers for Disease Control, August 14, 1987).

MEANING OF THE TEST

What Do Test Results Reveal?

A *true-positive* antibody test result (on the confirming Western blot test) means that the tested person is infected with the virus and may become sick at some time in the future and that the person can infect others by exchange of blood, semen, or vaginal fluid. A *true-negative* test means that a person is not infected. Other reasons for a negative test could be that the person is developing an immune response but not enough antibody has been produced to show up on a test, or that the person may have an unusual condition that prevents the immune system from developing antibodies.

What Do Tests Results Not Reveal?

The CDC has defined the presence of HIV antibodies as indicative of infection with HIV. All persons who are antibody positive should be considered infectious.

The test does *not* identify persons with AIDS or other HIV-related conditions. These conditions are only diagnosed when a person's case history matches a set of clinical signs and symptoms recognized by the CDC.

The percentage of persons with HIV antibodies who will develop AIDS is unknown. And since the test is designed to test only for antibodies to the virus, it does not identify all blood containing the virus.

A person who has been infected but has not had time to develop antibodies will test negative but is indeed infected and infectious. This person will test positive later, when the blood has developed significant numbers of antibodies.

Some people will test positive who are truly not infected. This unfortunate error, a false-positive result, may be caused by technician error or by a medical condition that makes the blood react positively to the antibody test.

In summary, although the test is very useful in identifying HIV-infected blood, it cannot predict which people will become sick, and it cannot identify people who are infected but for one reason or another are not producing antibodies to the virus.

TESTING ISSUES

Do-It-Yourself Test Kits

Some companies are offering do-it-yourself tests for people who want to test their own blood at home. These tests are prohibited by the Food and Drug Administration and should not be used.

Informed Consent for Testing

A person's informed consent should be obtained before his or her blood is tested for HIV antibody. In many states specific informed consent for HIV testing is required by law, and other states are considering such legislation. The goal of consent legislation is to be sure that patients choose to take the test only after knowing what the result may mean to them personally, medically, and socially.

The American Hospital Association states that testing for HIV infection is appropriately performed for the purposes of:

- Making a diagnosis of AIDS or ARC
- Answering a patient's question about whether he or she is infected
- Screening blood, organs, or other body substances prior to donation
- Conducting follow-up after a potential exposure to HIV has occurred (for example, after needle-stick injury or other inadvertent violation of universal precautions), whether the exposed person is a patient or an employee (AHA Report, 1987–88)

Although verbal consent is legally sufficient in most states, written consent is more easily proven in case of disputes and should be obtained. The patient's record should indicate when information or counseling has been given.

Physicians and hospitals are well advised to limit serum testing to instances where clinical need is well documented. This means that a physician should not assume that permission to draw blood for general clinical testing implies permission to administer an HIV antibody test. The physician should explain the medical purpose of the test, the possibility of inaccurate results, the ways in which test results may affect the patient's medical care, the range of personal considerations that may influence a person's decision to be tested, and other options the patient has for obtaining the test. The American Hospital Association has provided specific guidance on testing to hospitals and physicians in its publication, *AIDS Memorandum #3* (AHA, 1988).

Counseling

Many public health officials consider counseling the most important part of HIV antibody testing. Most states support the need for counseling persons before and after performing HIV antibody tests. The scarcity of trained counselors, however, has prevented some states from expanding their testing services (Rowe & Ryan, 1987).

Routine Testing

The CDC defines routine counseling and testing as the policy of providing these services to all clients, along with the information that testing will be performed. Except where testing is required by law, people have the right to decline testing without being denied health care or other services (Centers for Disease Control, August 14, 1987).

Routine testing for HIV antibodies is controversial because it raises questions about its benefits. Officials disagree about whether routine testing of certain groups would be a useful preventive measure, even when the test is combined with counseling and education. No state currently requires HIV antibody screening for the general population.

The CDC has recommended routine testing for:

- Persons seeking treatment for sexually transmitted disease in all health care settings, including the private physician's office
- IV drug users who are treated in any health care setting
- Persons who believe their behaviors put them at risk for disease
- Women of childbearing age who have identified risk factors for HIV infection
- Persons undergoing medical evaluation or treatment for clinical signs or symptoms associated with HIV
- Prostitutes

The CDC has also called for routine testing on a periodic basis of patients in hospitals (Centers for Disease Control, August 14, 1987). The American Hospital Association, however, does not recommend routine testing for patients or for hospital staff (AHA, 1987–88, p. iv) because HIV infection control practices should be standard operating procedure.

Compulsory Testing

Public health officials and some groups of citizens resist forced testing. Arguments against compulsory universal testing are: the expense is disproportionate to the benefit; it would likely be avoided by people who practice risky behaviors; and it would need to be repeated again and again on people who test negative.

Some states have begun to require that certain groups be screened. These groups include newborns in high-risk communities, prisoners, convicted prostitutes, all prostitutes in Nevada (the only state with legalized prostitution), and pregnant women with "high risk characteristics." Screening may be either anonymous or confidential.

One state (Illinois) has a law mandating premarital testing; other states provide HIV information with marriage license applications and alternate test sites for those who wish to be tested. The federal government requires that immigrants and people in the military or foreign service be tested.

Keeping Test Results Private

Confidential Testing

In confidential test sites, names and other identifying information are kept as part of a confidential patient record. Information is used only for public health purposes and is only available to authorized public health officials. States that require reporting of positive antibody status use confidential testing.

Anonymous Testing

In anonymous test sites, names and other identifying data are not collected, though information such as race and age may be recorded. Numbers are used to match test results with clients. Most states in which HIV test results are not reported to state or local health departments offer anonymous testing services. Some states permit a choice between anonymous and confidential testing.

It is generally believed that anonymity encourages people at high risk to obtain the test. Confidential testing, however, has the advantage of allowing officials to contact the person for follow-up testing or advice.

Testing Sites

Alternate Test Sites

When it became possible in March 1985 to test blood for HIV antibody, the federal government was concerned that people who knew they had practiced risky behaviors might donate blood in order to receive the test. If this were to happen on a large scale, some infected blood would get into the blood-banking system.

In order to protect the blood supply, the Centers for Disease Control funded what has become the Counseling and Testing Sites (CTS) program. This program has set up testing places in which people can receive anonymous or confidential testing without donating blood. Tests are provided at low or no cost. The sites are generally managed by a state, county, or local health department.

Private Physician's Office

Tests done in a private physician's office are not anonymous. They should be confidential but are not always. The cost of tests done in a physician's office generally ranges between $50 and $100.

EDUCATION FOR HEALTH CARE PROVIDERS ABOUT TESTING

Physicians and other health care providers are expected to determine who is at high risk of HIV infection and are required to counsel patients about testing or to assure that counseling is done by others. Physicians, nurses, and social workers who must make these decisions should receive education about legal responsibilities and how to identify individuals who should receive information.

SUMMARY

Of the many complex issues resulting from the AIDS epidemic, testing at present attracts the greatest public attention. The nature of the tests, the goals of public health, the rights of individuals, and value-laden political considerations all come together when public policy decisions must be made. What can be positively stated is that there are no simple answers. Policy makers are likely to proceed with caution as they begin to confront the implications of testing.

BIBLIOGRAPHY

American Hospital Association (1987–88). AIDS/HIV infection: recommendations for health care practices and public policy. *AHA Report,* p. iv. Chicago: American Hospital Association.

American Hospital Association (July, 1988). AIDS memorandum #3: HIV testing and informed consent. *AIDS Issues Update.* Chicago: American Hospital Association.

Centers for Disease Control (August 14, 1987). Public health service guidelines for counseling and antibody testing to prevent HIV infection and AIDS. *Morbidity and Mortality Weekly Report*: 509–515.

Curran, J. *et al.* (1985). The epidemiology of AIDS: Current status and future prospects. *Science,* 29:1352, 1354.

Dalton, H. L., S. Burris, & the Yale AIDS Law Project (eds.) (1987). AIDS and the Law: A Guide for the Public, p. 134. New Haven: Yale University Press.

Mann, D. L., C. Murray, R. Yarchoan, W. Blattner, & J. J. Goedert (1988). HLA antigen frequencies in HIV-1 seropositive disease-free individuals and patients with AIDS. *Journal of Acquired Immune Deficiency Syndromes, 1*(1):13–17.

Rowe, M., & C. Ryan (October, 1987). AIDS, A Public Health Challenge. Vol. 1. Assessing the Problem, pp. 2–37. Washington, DC: U.S. Department of Health and Human Services.

4

PUBLIC ISSUES
RELATED TO AIDS

This chapter discusses societal, ethical, and legal issues that are related to AIDS and HIV infection and that affect the lives and the practice of health care providers.

In the short period of less than a decade during which AIDS has become part of the public consciousness and conscience in the United States, individuals have acted ethically and unethically, legally and illegally, with personal courage and cowardice, with selflessness and selfishness.

People have had to face their fear of death. They have faced fears of homosexuality and of drug use and users. Perhaps most frightening of all, they have faced the fact that our highly praised, sophisticated medical care system can be "outwitted" by a seemingly elusive organism.

AIDS, or HIV, is only a part of the picture. The virus occurs in particular people, and those people have a legal right not to be discriminated against. Other people who don't have the disease don't want to catch it and have a right to protect themselves and their families.

SOCIETAL ISSUES

The major societal issues surrounding AIDS involve a real or perceived conflict between, on the one hand, the rights of infected people (or those considered infected) to privacy and equal access to housing, hospitalization, employment, and education and, on the other hand, rights of uninfected people to protect themselves against HIV and AIDS. Protection, in the context of AIDS, includes the right to know how the disease is spread. Major issues faced by society today include fear of the disease and of those who have it, education for prevention of infection, testing for the presence of HIV, and responsibility for caring for the sick.

Attitudes of people toward others are at the heart of the societal issues related to this epidemic. Apparent sources of negative attitudes of health care providers toward patients who are, or may be, HIV positive include fear of contagion and fear or dislike of homosexuals (homophobia) (Barrick, 1988). Negative attitudes may also come from care providers' inability to manage their own anger and fear associated with death or to alter the ultimate course of the disease.

Fears: Rational and Irrational

Fears about AIDS and HIV infection have both rational and irrational aspects. Important in the context of the AIDS epidemic are society's beliefs about and attitudes toward homosexuals, users of illegal drugs, and members of minority racial and ethnic groups. Attitudes toward death and disability are also important, particularly the death and disability of previously healthy young people.

It is rational to be afraid of AIDS. AIDS kills people. It is also rational to accept accurate information about transmission of HIV, to understand that the virus is not easily passed from one person to another, and to avoid behaviors that are known to increase the risk of infection. A rational fear can be managed. Irrational fear is the fear that remains when an informed person feels panic upon touching or even being in the same room with a person infected with the virus. Irrational fear is sometimes cured by getting to know a person with the virus or the disease, by shaking hands with or even hugging that person.

Beyond their fear, health care providers sometimes have an ethical problem related to dealing with people whom society values little or not at all. In regard to AIDS, there seems to be a set of attitudes that interferes with providing quality care.

Homophobia

Homophobia, or the fear of homosexuality, has become widespread as homosexual people have increasingly "come out of the closet." Fear of gays and lesbians has led to a variety of discriminatory acts from social snubbing to murder. Discrimination against homosexuals by health care providers has been associated with poor-quality health care. A health care provider who recognizes that this fear prevents the delivery of high-quality care may need to obtain information and assistance from self-help groups or from a professional.

Fear of Drug Use and Drug Users

Patients with AIDS include a high percentage of intravenous drug users. These people generally do not get medical attention early because they don't seek it and are sometimes shunned by care-providing systems. They are therefore likely to be very sick when they finally seek care. Often victims of addiction are malnourished, dirty, disheveled, and demanding.

It is not necessary to like a patient personally or to approve of his or her behavior to provide care. Everyone is entitled to the best possible care. There has been an attitude in our society that drug users deserve AIDS. This unfortunate perspective is unethical and shortsighted; it must be overcome in order to meet effectively the many health care needs of HIV-positive people and to provide education in prevention.

Racial Discrimination

As of November 1988, 26 percent of AIDS cases had occurred among blacks and 15 percent among Latinos. These percentages are higher than the percentages those groups represent in the general United States population. Among children with AIDS, 53 percent are black and 23 percent are Latino.

Education

The Public Health Service has asserted that prevention is the only effective means of controlling AIDS at present.

Now, and for the foreseeable future, education is the means by which prevention will be achieved; lives can be saved by education.

The need for education, however, raises controversial issues about the proper content of an AIDS educational program, the proper age at which to begin the program, and the groups to be targeted for education. Educational issues include the societal dilemma as to whether sex education is the responsibility of the family or a public necessity. Other concerns involve effective methods of educating intravenous drug users.

Sex Education for Young People

Medical experts agree that certain sexual practices are not likely to spread HIV infection. These include masturbating alone and dry kissing. If no semen or blood is present, body-to-body rubbing, mutual masturbation, massage, hugging, and using clean sex toys that are not shared are also relatively safe practices.

Experts also agree that certain other sexual practices may spread the disease: intercourse of any kind (rectal, vaginal, oral) where there is an exchange of blood, semen, or vaginal fluid, "rimming" (placing a tongue in the rectum of a partner), "fisting" (placing a hand in the rectum of a partner) if exchange of semen or blood follows.

Although there is agreement about relatively safe and unsafe sexual practices, there is no general consensus on how to talk, especially to young people, about these and other sexual behaviors. A great many people believe that sex education promotes sexual activity, which they would rather discourage.

The Condom Debate

There is no doubt that the spread of HIV infection could be better curtailed by increased use of condoms and other barrier devices during sexual activities. Yet education about condoms is opposed by those who disapprove of birth control (a major purpose of condoms) and of homosexuality.

The effectiveness of condoms in preventing disease is related to the quality of the condom and to the technique used in applying it and keeping it in place. Instructions on how to use a condom are provided in Chapter 2.

Clean Drug Paraphernalia

There is also no question that the best way to prevent infection is not to use drugs in the first place. This simplistic answer will not work in the short run, however, and perhaps not in the long run either. The goal of preventing the spread of a deadly disease needs to take precedence over preventing drug abuse, as worthy as the latter goal is.

Making clean needles available and teaching drug users how to clean used ones would unquestionably help to curb the spread of HIV infection. Instructions on how to clean needles are provided in Chapter 2.

Testing

Testing issues generally revolve around the conflict between the rights of the individual over his or her own body and the right of the public to be protected from a deadly disease. Testing issues are discussed in Chapter 3.

The Cost of Providing Care to Affected Persons

AIDS is a very expensive illness. Average lifetime hospital costs range from $60,000 to $75,000 per case. By 1991 AIDS medical care costs could be $16 billion or higher.

State Medicaid programs bear, nationally, 25 percent ($400 million in 1987) of the medical costs of AIDS. This does not include costs associated with providing the drug, AZT, which was estimated to have reached $150 million in 1988 (Carbine & Lee, 1988, pp. 15–16).

The very sickest patients need skilled, and often continuous, intensive care. Who will provide the care? In what settings? Care in the home is considerably less expensive than hospital care, but home care of the type needed is not presently available in many communities. The cost of the development of new medications will be staggering. It is certain that these costs must be born by society, but how the costs will be apportioned will be debated in the legislatures.

ETHICAL ISSUES

There is a difference between *morality* and *ethics*. As used in this discussion, moral behavior conforms to custom or tradition. Ethical behavior, on the other hand, is the result of a considered, rational decision about right and wrong. In a particular situation it may or may not be the same as moral behavior; the ethical decision is above, or beyond, merely moral behavior.

Professional Associations and Ethics

The American Medical Association and the American Nurses' Association have ethical codes meant to guide the behavior of their members. (See box for American Nurses' Association Codes for Nurses.) The American Medical Association (AMA), in its 1980 *Principles of Medical Ethics,* states:

> A physician shall respect the rights of patients, of colleagues, and of other health professionals, and shall safeguard patient confidences within the constraints of the law.

In addition, the AMA Council on Ethical and Judicial Affairs has stated that a physician may not ethically refuse to treat a patient whose condition is within the physician's realm of competence solely because the patient is seropositive for antibody to HIV (Council on Ethical and Judicial Affairs, 1988, p. 1360).

LEGAL ISSUES

Refusing to Give Care

Professional health care providers should not refuse care. Medical students, nurses, nursing students, and

AMERICAN NURSES' ASSOCIATION
CODE FOR NURSES

The Code for Nurses is based upon belief about the nature of individuals, nursing, health, and society. Recipients and providers of nursing services are viewed as individuals and groups who possess basic rights and responsibilities, and whose values and circumstances command respect at all times. Nursing encompasses the promotion and restoration of health, the prevention of illness, and the alleviation of suffering. *The statements of the Code and their interpretation provide guidance for conduct and relationships in carrying out nursing responsibilities consistent with the ethical obligations of the profession and quality in nursing care.*

- The nurse provides services with respect for human dignity and the uniqueness of the client unrestricted by considerations of social or economic status, personal attributes, or the nature of health problems.
- The nurse safeguards the client's right to privacy by judiciously protecting information of a confidential nature.
- The nurse acts to safeguard the client and the public when health care and safety are affected by the incompetent, unethical, or illegal practice of any person.
- The nurse assumes responsibility and accountability for individual nursing judgments and actions.
- The nurse maintains competence in nursing.
- The nurse exercises informed judgment and uses individual competence and qualifications as criteria in seeking consultation, accepting responsibilities, and delegating nursing activities to others.
- The nurse participates in activities that contribute to the ongoing development of the profession's body of knowledge.
- The nurse participates in the profession's efforts to implement and improve standards of nursing.
- The nurse participates in the profession's efforts to establish and maintain conditions of employment conducive to high-quality nursing care.
- The nurse participates in the profession's effort to protect the public from misinformation and misrepresentation and to maintain the integrity of nursing.
- The nurse collaborates with members of the health professions and other citizens in promoting community and national efforts to meet the health needs of the public.

Reprinted with permission of American Nurses' Association. (1985). Code for Nurses with Interpretive Statements. 2420 Pershing Road, Kansas City, MO 64108: American Nurses' Association.

CODE OF ETHICS FOR THE
LICENSED PRACTICAL NURSE

- The licensed practical nurse shall practice her profession with integrity.
- The licensed practical nurse shall be loyal—to the physician, to the patient, and to her employer.
- The licensed practical nurse strives to know her limitations and to stay within the bounds of these limitations.
- The licensed practical nurse is sincere in the performance of her duties and generous in rendering service.
- The licensed practical nurse considers no duty too menial if it contributes to the welfare and comfort of her patient.
- The licensed practical nurse accepts only that monetary compensation which is provided for in the contract under which she is employed, and she does not solicit gifts.
- The licensed practical nurse holds in confidence all information entrusted to her.
- The licensed practical nurse shall be a good citizen.
- The licensed practical nurse participates in and shares responsibility for meeting health needs.
- The licensed practical nurse faithfully carries out the orders of the physician or registered nurse under whom she serves.
- The licensed practical nurse refrains from entering into conversation with the patient about personal experiences, personal problems, and personal ailments.

Reprinted with permission of American Nurses' Association. (1985). Code for Nurses with Interpretive Statements. 2420 Pershing Road, Kansas City, MO 64108: American Nurses' Association.

other people employed by or being trained within the hospital to provide care are obligated to treat all patients admitted by the hospital (Banks, 1987).

Right to Know

Professional Nurses

Nurses sometimes believe they can only give good, holistic care when they know all there is to know about a client; but some clients choose not to share personal information. The answer to the question of whether or not health care providers have a right to know whether a patient is HIV positive—in general—is no. The Centers for Disease Control (CDC) has issued guidelines for universal precautions so that it is not necessary to know whether a particular person's blood is seropositive for HIV.

While some state laws allow information about the HIV status of a patient to be given to a patient's health care providers, recent guidelines from the Occupational Safety and Health Administration (OSHA) state that OSHA's hazard communication standard (Employee's Right-to-Know) only applies to chemical or physical hazards in the workplace; it does not apply to biologic hazards such as blood-borne disease (U.S. Department of Labor, OSHA, August 1988).

Other Care Providers

The question may arise as to whether nursing assistants, ward clerks, housekeeping staff, and other health agency employees have a right to know anyone's HIV status. All health care agency employees should assume that all patients and personal acquaintances are potentially HIV positive and that all people have a right to keep information about their HIV status private. They should be given these instructions and told that if they attempt to violate the confidentiality policy of the employing agency, they may be released from employment.

Sexual Partners of
HIV-Positive Persons

Issues involving notification of sexual partners are especially controversial. Sexual partners apparently do have a right to know each other's HIV status (Davis, 1988). A physician to whom sexual partners of an HIV-positive patient have been identified probably has a personal duty to disclose the patient's HIV status to them if, and only if, attempts to encourage voluntary disclosure have failed (Council on Ethical and Judicial Affairs, 1988, pp. 1360–61). However, the U.S. House of Representatives rejected legislation *requiring* doctors to inform spouses of AIDS patients about the patients' positive status (*New York Times,* September 17, 1988).

Malpractice

Only those health care providers who practice under a professional license are subject to malpractice action. Others may be prosecuted for negligence—a breach of duty reasonably owed by any person in the situation.

Malpractice is professional negligence and acknowledges a higher duty of a licensed professional to a patient than the usual duty of one layperson to another. In a malpractice case, the person bringing charges (the plaintiff) must show that "there is more evidence than not" that four conditions existed at the time of the incident:

- The defendant owed a duty to the client.
- The defendant breached that duty in some way.
- Some damage resulted to the client.
- The defendant caused the damage.

The breach of duty may be something the professional *did* or something he or she *did not do* but should have done. Standards of practice help to establish what a reasonably prudent professional would have done under the same or similar circumstances. Such standards include relevant federal laws, state laws including state practice acts, and rules and regulations of licensing boards. Various published professional standards and ethical codes may also establish prevailing standards, although these documents are not "laws."

Sanctions

A variety of sanctions can be imposed upon a practitioner for not meeting legal, ethical, or practice standards. A professional association, such as the American Nurses' Association, may sanction by expulsion from membership in the association. State boards of nursing in all 50 states may remove a license "for cause." Actions of nurses that have caused removal include unethical conduct as well as conviction in a criminal case.

Determining Potential
for Successful Legal Action

Health care providers can be sued for irresponsible professional behavior. The success or failure of the suit depends on many factors. Patients sue primarily because they are angry or frustrated. The best defense against litigation, therefore, is to maintain good relationships with patients. Other preventive actions include maintaining skills and documenting the care given to patients.

Potential Legal Actions

Potential legal actions in connection with AIDS and HIV infection include actions that may be brought by patients, families, and co-workers against a health care provider (individual or agency), actions against employers by health care providers, and actions against licensed health care providers by licensing boards.

Suits Against Health Care Providers

Suits by Patients or Co-workers for Breach of Confidentiality. The only reason to break confidentiality concerning a particular patient's condition would be that a health care provider believed that a *known* third party was in unwitting danger of contracting the disease. The specific health care provider responsible for making this disclosure, if anyone is, is the *patient's primary provider—usually the physician in charge of the case.* The identifiability of the potential victim is an important factor for most courts; if the victim is unknown, the courts have ruled in favor of the allegedly dangerous client (Belitsky & Solomon, 1987).

Suit by a Patient Alleging That a Health Care Provider Didn't Take Proper Precautions (According to Hospital Policy) and Thus Transmitted the Disease Either from the Provider or from Another Patient. As patients begin to expect that precautions will be used to protect them as well as to protect health care providers, it becomes important to use such precautions consistently. A patient who believes that he or she has acquired an infection in the hospital could bring legal action.

Suit by a Patient or Family Alleging That the Provider Didn't Act Quickly Enough in an Emergency Because of Inappropriate Fear of Contracting Disease from the Patient. Certain actions, such as carrying out a "slow code" order (where the health care provider purposely acts slowly to institute life-saving measures), put a patient's life in jeopardy and have no legitimate basis. If a patient does not wish to have extraordinary measures performed, the physician is obligated to write this request in the form of an "order" in the patient's medical chart. Lacking the written order, the health care provider must respond with vigor to an emergency.

Since the response of the provider should be independent of any actual or possible disease process in the patient, protective equipment and clothing should be easily accessible in all patient care areas. Some health care providers carry small plastic mouth protectors so that they will not waste precious time when mouth-to-mouth resuscitation is needed.

Suits Against Hospitals

Suit Against a Hospital or Other Employing Health Care Agency by a Nurse Who Becomes HIV Positive.   A health care provider who becomes HIV positive after an accidental exposure to blood would be able to recover damages only if the hospital or agency had not met its legal obligations to the worker. These obligations are discussed in detail in Chapter 6.

Suit Against a Hospital or Other Employing Agency by a Nurse Who Has Been Fired for Refusing to Care for Clients Who Are HIV Positive.   While an employer hospital can fire an employee (especially when the employee is not covered by a union contract) whose refusal to give care is based on irrational fear, the hospital would serve all interests better by providing education and opportunities for the employee to overcome fear. Discharging employees because of their panic reactions does not seem an effective way to deal with a situation that might settle down with appropriate efforts at employee education (Leonard, 1987). However, if reasonable efforts to educate fail, the employing hospital is justified in terminating employment.

Suit Against a Hospital by a Patient Who Was Tested for Antibody to HIV Without Express Consent.   Several legal actions have claimed that a hospital violated its obligation to obtain informed consent before performing an HIV antibody test. Some states have specific legislation requiring informed consent for HIV testing; in states that have not passed such legislation, the American Hospital Association recommends obtaining specific, informed consent for the test (AHA, 1987–88, p. 12).

Actions by Licensing Boards

Removal of license for breach of ethics (breach of confidentiality or refusal to provide care) is the responsibility of each of the professional licensing boards. Every nurse should obtain a personal copy of the act governing nursing practice in his or her state.

HIV-Positive
Health Care Providers

In Chicago, the county board's Health and Hospitals Committee recently approved a recommendation that would allow Cook County Hospital patients the right to refuse to be treated by workers who "carry the AIDS virus" (*New York Times,* September 16, 1988, p. B-7). This recommendation runs counter to recommendations of all major professional and hospital associations and government agencies.

The federal laws most useful in helping HIV-positive health care providers to keep their jobs are those related to discrimination in employment of the handicapped. Section 504 of the United States Federal Rehabilitation Act of 1973 provides that "otherwise qualified handicapped individuals" may not be excluded from participation in, denied the benefits of, or subject to discrimination under any program or activity receiving federal financial assistance or conducted by any federal agency or the Postal Service. Several federal courts have ruled that Section 504 gives individuals the right to sue their employers for discrimination (Leonard, 1987).

State handicap laws may also be useful in states where the law expressly or by implication includes infectious disease as a handicap. These laws are meant to enhance employment opportunities for the handicapped. Of course, the laws protect only "otherwise qualified" individuals; those too sick to work or for whom "reasonable accommodation" cannot be made are not covered.

Another avenue of assistance, should a person actually lose a job, may be unemployment insurance. Leonard points out that "employees who are discharged solely because of their medical condition at a time when they are physically able to work are undoubtedly eligible for unemployment insurance benefits, since their discharges could not be said to be for 'just cause' or 'misbehavior' on the job, the usual bases of disqualification after an involuntary termination of employment" (Leonard, 1987). The same should be true of individuals—relatives or close friends of persons with HIV—who are not infected but who lose their jobs because of AIDS panic.

Discrimination Against
Health Care Providers

Unfortunately, discrimination against those who deal daily with HIV-positive patients, or with individuals considered by the public to be at risk for AIDS, has been a problem for some health care providers and their families. As the public becomes better informed, and as more people become HIV positive, the fear and discrimination will decrease.

SUMMARY

The issues that are emerging in this age of AIDS are global issues about how to assure that all persons are treated respectfully and justly. More than 250,000 cases of AIDS have already been reported worldwide, and between 5 and 10 million people have been infected with the virus (Mann *et al.*, 1988, p. 82). This disease and its horrible consequences will be with us for decades, if not for generations; the choices we make today on the issues will be important in influencing what happens to our country and to our world.

BIBLIOGRAPHY

American Hospital Association (1987–88). Report and recommendations for health care practices and public policy. *AHA Report.* Chicago: American Hospital Association.

American Medical Association (1980). Principles of medical ethics. Chicago: American Medical Association.

American Nurses' Association (1976). Code for nurses. Kansas City: American Nurses' Association.

Banks, T. L. (1987). The right to medical treatment. In H. L.

Dalton, & S. Burris (eds.), *AIDS and the Law*, p. 179. New Haven: Yale University Press.

Barrick, B. (1988). The willingness of nursing personnel to care for patients with acquired immune deficiency syndrome: A survey study and recommendations. *Journal of Professional Nursing, 4*(5), 366–372.

Belitsky, R., & R. A. Solomon (1987). Doctors and patients: Responsibilities in a confidential relationship. In H. L. Dalton, & S. Burris (eds.), *AIDS and the Law*, p. 205. New Haven: Yale University Press.

Carbine, M. E., & P. Lee (1988). AIDS into the '90's: Strategies for an Integrated Response to the AIDS Epidemic. Washington, DC: National AIDS Network.

Council on Ethical and Judicial Affairs (1988). Ethical issues involved in the growing AIDS crisis. *Journal of the American Medical Association, 259*(9), 1360.

Davis, M. (1988). Lovers, Doctors & the Law. New York: Harper & Row.

House rejects bid to require disclosure to AIDS spouses (September 17, 1988). *New York Times.*

Leonard, A. S. (1987). AIDS in the workplace. In H. L. Dalton, & S. Burris (eds.), *AIDS and the Law*, pp. 109–125. New Haven: Yale University Press.

Mann, J. M., J. Chin, P. Piot, & T. Quinn (1988). The international epidemiology of AIDS. *Scientific American, 259*(4), 82–89.

Right to bar treatment by any with AIDS virus weighed (September 16, 1988). *New York Times.*

U.S. Department of Labor, Occupational Safety and Health Administration (August 1988). Instruction CPL 2-2.44A: Enforcement procedures for occupational exposure to hepatitis B virus (HBV) and human immunodeficiency virus (HIV). Washington, DC: U.S. Department of Labor.

5

COMMUNITY RESOURCES

This chapter discusses the ways in which federal and state governments, private organizations, and local communities can address problems resulting from HIV infection. A list of organizations, hotlines, and newsletters offering information and assistance is included at the end of the chapter.

FEDERAL GOVERNMENT

If AIDS is the number one health priority of the nation, as government officials have stated, how is that priority translated into policy, money, and action? In the United States, all three branches of government—legislative, administrative, and judicial—participate in an ongoing effort to combat disease and promote healthful practices. The United States Public Health Service was created by Congress—the *legislative* branch of government—and is responsible to it. Through its research divisions, the National Institutes of Health (NIH) and the Centers for Disease Control (CDC), disease is studied both in patients (by the NIH) and in the laboratory (by the CDC).

The *administration* sets policy through cabinet officials who direct regulatory agencies. In dealing with AIDS, the two most important cabinet officials are the Secretary for Health and Human Services, who heads the Department of Health and Human Services (DHHS), and the Secretary of Education, who heads the Department of Education (DOE).

The *judicial* system attempts to maintain consistency in major decisions by setting and following precedents and by assuring that current laws fall within the general guidelines provided by the United States Constitution.

United States
Public Health Service (USPHS)

The Public Health Service (PHS), one of four operating units of DHHS, has six components, all of which are of critical importance in the country's efforts to curb the AIDS epidemic. These components are:

- Alcohol, Drug Abuse and Mental Health Administration
- Centers for Disease Control
- Food and Drug Administration
- Health Resources and Services Administration
- National Institutes of Health
- Agency for Toxic Substances and Disease Registry

Roles of the Surgeon General and
the Secretary for Education

The Surgeon General of the United States deals with *prevention of disease*. When prevention is clearly related to behaviors that can only be affected by education and individual decision making, then the Surgeon General must also deal with education. The Surgeon General issued the *Report on Acquired Immune Deficiency Syndrome* in 1986 and *Understanding AIDS* in 1988.

The primary responsibility for general *education* and for the publication of national education policy rests with the Department of Education, whose secretary, unlike the Surgeon General, is a member of the president's cabinet. This administrative position is subject to political pressures and constraints that the Surgeon General may be able to ignore.

The persons holding the positions of Surgeon General and of Secretary for Education must represent public views rather than their personal opinions. Surgeon General C. Everett Koop has said that no matter what his personal opinions about proper sexual behavior, his job is to advise the public in such a way as to prevent disease. The Secretary for Education is not under public mandate to prevent disease; his primary job is to suggest educational policy that is in line with the prevailing values of the elected administration.

The AIDS epidemic has produced a conflict between these two efforts. Educating for disease prevention requires the use of sexually explicit words and open discussion of sexual behaviors that many people regard as inappropriate. At the heart of the issue is the unanswered question whether talking about controversial activities gives those activities a stamp of approval or whether free discussion helps people to make rational, health-promoting choices in the expression of their sexuality and need for intimacy.

STATE GOVERNMENT

Attempts to control the AIDS epidemic are undertaken primarily at the state and local levels of government. Following is a list of important activities of state governments related to the control of HIV infection:

- Protect public health
- Direct public education
- License and regulate health care professionals
- Provide access to medical care for people unable to afford it
- Regulate insurers, who influence access to costly health services
- Provide civil legal protection where federal statutes leave gaps
- Translate policies into programs to meet the day-to-day needs of patients, their families, friends, and health care providers

An excellent resource for those concerned with state issues regarding AIDS is the three-volume Public Health Services document, *AIDS: A Public Health Challenge, State Issues, Policies and Programs* (Rowe & Ryan, 1987).

PRIVATE ORGANIZATIONS

Private charitable organizations and foundations have funded a variety of efforts to control HIV infection.

Private health care organizations such as the American Red Cross have developed community-based AIDS education programs. Organizations such as Gay Men's Health Crisis in New York are at the forefront of efforts to provide social services to people with AIDS, including legal assistance, self-help groups, and direct care.

LOCAL COMMUNITY

In many communities, AIDS councils or task forces have been established to coordinate and direct efforts to combat the disease at the community level. A partial list of public and private organizations is presented at the end of this chapter.

A community, no matter what its size, can mobilize to meet the challenge of the AIDS epidemic. (See box for list of resources communities might bring to bear upon the problem.) Categories commonly used in talking about the disease (AIDS, ARC, HIV infection without symptoms) are identified and types of resources needed to solve the more obvious problems are presented. This model can be used to identify organizations that should be included in long-range planning for effective community action against AIDS.

Involving Groups

Following is a list of the kinds of organizations that can be involved in specific planning efforts to deal with the AIDS epidemic in a community.

- Racial and ethnic minority organizations
- Family planning organizations
- Gay and lesbian organizations
- Religious groups
- Hospital and nursing home representatives
- Hospices
- Home care providers
- Health care providers—physicians, dentists, nurses, dietitians, physical therapists
- Epidemiologists

**COMMUNITY NEED FOR SERVICES
RELATED TO HIV INFECTION**

AIDS (cases by CDC definition)
- Hospital beds
- Intensive care (nurses, respiratory therapists, physicians)
- Hospices
- Home care
- Spiritual guidance
- Meal delivery programs
- AIDS support groups
- Counseling services

ARC (AIDS-related complex)
- Clinic facilities (physicians, laboratories, nurses)
- Schools
- News media (print, radio, TV)
- AIDS support groups
- AIDS information hotline
- Residence support

HIV-positive persons without symptoms
Diagnostic facilities (public health dept., private labs)
Educators, for prevention of irrational fear and to teach behaviors that will limit spread among:
- IV drug abusers
- Prisoners in prison and after release
- Prostitutes
- Sexual contacts of prostitutes
- Young, sexually active individuals
- Young children at risk of sexual abuse by persons with HIV infection
- Abused women, men, and children

Noninfected public
Educators (targeting services to specific needs of individuals and groups)
Education should be:
- Individualized
- Nonjudgmental
- Updated as new information becomes available
- Culture sensitive
- Ethnically appropriate

- Public health department
- Police department
- Colleges, universities
- Technical and trade schools
- Prisons
- Media (print, radio, television)
- Restaurants
- Primary and secondary schools
- American Red Cross
- Legal experts
- Women's resource centers
- Health planning organizations
- Drug rehabilitation centers
- Social workers, social work educators
- Health educators
- Insurance industry representatives
- Organizations for the homeless
- Legislators
- Labor organizations

Community-Based AIDS Task Force

Recognizing the variety of services needed and the variety of groups that should be involved in a campaign to manage the social, medical, educational, and legal problems presented by this disease, many communities have developed an AIDS task force. Complimenting the medical, psychological, and social networks already in place, such a group can often obtain funding that is not available to individuals working alone. A group spokesperson can address emotional issues concerning HIV infection in an accurate, reasoned public voice.

The task force has the advantage of including representation from many disciplines, professions, and interest groups. A critical element in assuring its success is the leader's ability to incorporate the expertise of members into a unified vision—and to move the group to action.

Responsibilities

The responsibilities of a community AIDS task force could include:

1. Identify Community Strengths.   In most communities some activities related to AIDS are already underway. In addition, every community has experts in some aspect of AIDS treatment, education, or prevention or in community organization.

2. Identify Community Needs.   Programs developed to care for HIV-positive persons or to prevent infection need to have access to critical information in order to set reasonable goals. They will need epidemiologic data concerning the incidence of HIV infection in the community, information about the level of understanding about HIV infection and the use of risk-reduction strategies among individuals, and the current practices of health care providers in the community.

3. Set Initial Goals.   A set of priority goals can be developed after an initial assessment of needs. Goals that some communities have set include:

- Develop an ongoing media education campaign geared to prevent panic.
- Educate groups known to present the highest risk of transmission (homosexual or bisexual men and users of intravenous drugs).
- Develop an AIDS hotline.
- Obtain local community consensus on curricular materials for kindergarten through grade 12.
- Develop support groups for patients and families.
- Provide housing for homeless patients.

4. Identify Needed Resources.   The group may seek initial support for its efforts from private foundations in the area or from various citizens' groups. The group might elect a governing board, identify sources of income, set up an office, and hire staff—or it might manage its activities totally through the work of volunteers. The USPHS has issued guidelines that can be used to develop community-based AIDS prevention programs (Centers for Disease Control, October 1987).

5. Identify Constraints. Once goals and needed resources are identified, a list of constraints should be developed. Constraints might include not only a lack of money, space, and expertise, but also problems of intense fear and panic, which block rational thinking.

6. Set Criteria for Evaluation. It is essential for continued success and continued funding that group members decide how they will know when a goal has been achieved. Failure to conduct an ongoing evaluation will inevitably result in inefficient use of resources, frustration, confusion, and conflict among members.

Hospital AIDS
Volunteer Programs

In the wake of the AIDS epidemic, an unusual response has been seen among those who work with AIDS clients in hospitals—hospital-based AIDS volunteer programs. There are no blueprints for making such a program work well in a particular community. However, an article in the journal, *AIDS Patient Care,* details the experiences of several hospitals in recruiting, training, and retaining volunteers to serve in this new effort (Sears, 1988).

SUMMARY

While both federal and state governments are engaged in efforts to combat the epidemic, private organizations and groups of citizens have taken on a moral obligation to address issues of HIV infection in their own communities. As one hotline volunteer said, "If I can help to keep just one person from becoming infected, I will feel like the effort is worth it." This spirit, when adopted by hundreds of thousands of citizens, most certainly will help to stop the advance of this dread disease.

SOURCES FOR HELP

Information Sources

- AIDS Action Council
  729 Eighth Street SE, Suite 200
  Washington, DC 20003
  Phone: (202) 547-3101

- American Association of Physicians for Human Rights
  P.O. Box 14366
  San Francisco, CA 94114
  Phone: (415) 558-9353

- American College Health Association
  15879 Crabbs Branch Way
  Rockville, MD 20855
  Phone: (301) 963-1100

- American Dental Association
  211 East Chicago Avenue, Suite 2100
  Chicago, IL 60611
  Phone: (312) 440-2886

- American Hospital Association
  50 F Street NW, Suite 1100
  Washington, DC 20001
  Phone: (202) 638-1100

- American Medical Association
  1101 Vermont Avenue NW
  Washington, DC 20005
  Phone: (202) 789-7400

- American Nurses' Association
  1101 14th St. NW, Suite 200
  Washington, DC 20005
  Phone: (202) 789-1800

- American Red Cross
  AIDS Education Office
  1730 D Street NW
  Washington, DC 20006
  Phone: (202) 737-8300

- Gay Men's Health Crisis
  P.O. Box 274
  132 West 24th Street
  New York, NY 10011
  Phone: (212) 807-6655

- Hispanic AIDS Forum c/o APRED
  853 Broadway, Suite 2007
  New York, NY 10003
  Phone: (212) 870-1902 or 870-1864

- Los Angeles AIDS Project
  1362 Santa Monica Boulevard
  Los Angeles, CA 90046
  Phone: (213) 871-AIDS

- Minority Task Force on AIDS
  c/o New York City Council of Churches
  475 Riverside Drive, Room 456
  New York, NY 10115
  Phone: (212) 749-1214

- Mothers of AIDS Patients (MAP)
  Barbara Peabody
  3403 E Street
  San Diego, CA 29102
  Phone: (610) 234-3432

- National AIDS Network
  729 Eighth Street SE, Suite 300
  Washington, DC 20003
  Phone: (202) 546-2424

- National Association of People with AIDS
  P.O. Box 65472
  Washington, DC 20035
  Phone: (202) 483-7979

- National Coalition of Gay Sexually Transmitted
    Disease Services
  c/o Mark Behar
  P.O. Box 239
  Milwaukee, WI 53201
  Phone: (414) 277-7671

- National Council of Churches AIDS Task Force
  475 Riverside Drive, Room 472
  New York, NY 10115
  Phone: (212) 870-2421

- National Hemophilia Foundation
  110 Greene Street, Room 406
  New York, NY 10012
  Phone: (212) 219-8180

- San Francisco AIDS Foundation
  333 Valencia Street 4th Floor
  San Francisco, CA 94103
  Phone: (415) 863-2437

- SHANTI Project
  525 Howard Street
  San Francisco, CA 94105
  Phone: (415) 777-CARE

- VOLUNTEER: The National Center
  1111 North 19th, Suite 500
  Arlington, VA 22209
  Phone: (703) 276-0541

Hotlines
- US PHS AIDS Hotline
  1-800-342-AIDS
  1-800-342-2437

- AIDS Information Clearing House
  1-800-458-5231

- National Sexually Transmitted Diseases Hotline
  American Social Health Association
  1-800-227-8922

- National Gay Task Force AIDS Information Hotline
  1-800-221-7044
  In New York, (212) 807-6016

- Drug Abuse Help
  AIDS Information
  1-800-662-HELP

- AZT (Azidothymidine) Questions
  1-800-843-9388

AIDS Newsletters and Journals

AIDS Alert.   Monthly update on AIDS for health care professionals. Published by:

American Health Consultants, Inc.
Department 4651
67 Peachtree Park Drive NE
Atlanta, Georgia 30309

AIDS Weekly Surveillance Report.   United States Program, Center for Infectious Diseases, Centers for Disease Control (CDC). Provides a weekly update on the number of AIDS cases reported to the CDC. For information: (404) 329-3286

AIDS Patient Care: A Magazine for Health Care Professionals
Mary Ann Liebert, Inc.
1651 Third Avenue
New York, NY 10128
(212) 289-2300

BIBLIOGRAPHY

Centers for Disease Control (1987). Guidelines for AIDS Prevention Program Operations (DHHS Publications No. 00-5104). Washington, DC: Department of Health and Human Services.

Centers for Disease Control (1988). Understanding AIDS. U.S. Department of Health and Human Services.

Koop, C. E. (1986). Surgeon General's Report on Acquired Immune Deficiency Syndrome. Washington, DC: U.S. Public Health Service.

Rowe, M., & C. Ryan (October 1987). AIDS: A Public Health Challenge, 3 Vols. Washington, DC: U.S. Department of Health and Human Services.

Sears, C. (1988). Volunteers: How to get them, train them, and keep them. *AIDS Patient Care, 2*(4): 18–20.

6

OBLIGATIONS
OF THE EMPLOYER

This chapter discusses the responsibilities of the employer to the health care provider and to the patient with respect to protection against HIV infection. Legislative and regulatory origins of these obligations are reviewed.

OBLIGATIONS TO PROVIDERS

The employer has a duty to provide all employees with protective apparel and equipment, information about protection and transmission, policies for disposal of needles and sharp instruments that are consistent with accepted standards, policies about confidentiality in patient care situations, procedures to be followed in the case of a potentially infectious incident, monitoring of compliance with infection control policies, the assurance that employees' health and other records remain confidential, and nondiscriminatory employment.

Protective Apparel and Equipment

It is the legal responsibility of employers to provide appropriate safeguards for health care workers who may be exposed to blood-borne infection. The Occupational Safety and Health Administration (OSHA) and the Department of Labor direct employers to classify all work-related tasks into three categories: tasks that always require protective equipment or apparel (Category I), tasks that *may* require such equipment and apparel (Category II), and tasks that do not require protective apparel or equipment (Category III) (U.S. Department of Labor/Department of Health and Human Services, October 30, 1987). OSHA has set precise standards of quality for apparel, equipment, and disposal containers (U.S. Department of Labor, August 1988). These standards carry the force of federal law, and violation of them would place a health care agency at risk for fines or other disciplinary measures.

Apparel usually made available to health care providers includes gowns, gloves, goggles, and masks. Equipment includes disposable respiratory supplies, needle disposal units, and garbage bags. As noted, there is a clear duty of the employing agency, deriving from federal regulations, to provide a protection program to limit exposure of a worker to infectious diseases of all kinds. Such programs are in place or are being developed within health care agencies at the present time.

Information on Protection and Transmission

An employer must be able to assert that an employed health care provider has the necessary knowledge to meet patient care standards, including standards related to infection control. To meet this obligation, the employer should make and document a reasonable effort to provide education. The American Hospital Association states that hospitals should provide basic education on HIV infection and AIDS to all staff and should provide more extensive, tailored training and periodic follow-up as appropriate (AHA, 1987–88).

A record of this education with updates, filed in the permanent record of the employee, provides evidence that the education was given. Instruction for health care workers who have patient contact should include how to protect other workers by taking particular care not to leave needles or other sharp objects in linens, drawers, or garbage bags.

Policies on Disposal of Needles and Other Sharp Instruments

Needle-sticks and punctures from sharp objects account for many of the accidents experienced by health care providers. It is important to pay strict attention to the safe disposal of these items. Some hospitals, nursing homes, and home care agencies retain a policy of recapping needles after use, clearly violating the statement in the CDC guidelines: "Do not recap used needles by hand; do not remove used needles from disposable syringes by hand; and do not bend, break or otherwise manipulate used needles by hand" (Centers for Disease Control, June 24, 1988). The reuse of a disposable plastic sleeve used in drawing blood is another risky procedure that is in common practice in some home care agencies and hospitals.

An agency adopting a policy that does not provide for safe needle treatment is at legal risk of suit by an injured employee or patient because, although the risk of infection from an occupational exposure is small, the consequences of HIV infection can be extremely serious. Health care agencies must provide sufficient high-quality collection containers for needles and other sharp items. Similarly, an agency falls below patient care standards if it does not monitor employee actions to assure compliance with its policies.

Confidentiality in Patient Care Situations

Rowe and Ryan state that "employers must notify workers if they are handling the tissues or body fluids of patients who may be infected with an infectious organism if the handling of such infectious samples is not an everyday practice" (Rowe & Ryan, 1987, pp. 4–18). In August 1988, however, OSHA issued a directive (29 CFR 1910.1200), stating that the employee's right-to-know only applies to hazardous chemicals or physical hazards in the workplace, and thus does not apply to biological hazards such as blood-borne diseases (U.S. Department of Labor, August 1988). Health care providers are best advised to use universal precautions in all direct contact with patients or with laboratory specimens.

Incidents of Exposure

The employer must provide policies and procedures for employees who have been exposed to blood on the job through needle-stick injuries or through extensive mucous membrane exposure. The policies should include:

- A definition of "high risk"
- Assignment of responsibility for paying for HIV antibody tests
- A schedule for testing
- Assignment of responsibility for providing counseling for the exposed person
- Assignment of responsibility for obtaining informed consent of both parties for testing
- Assurance of confidentiality of test results, the exposure occurrence, and testing

Monitoring Compliance with Infection Control Policies

The American Hospital Association stresses the obligation of the employer to monitor compliance with standards of infection control among health care providers in the institution. They point out that compliance monitoring and enforcement are, ultimately, in the best interest of all hospital staff (AHA, 1987–88).

Confidentiality Regarding Health Records and Evaluation Data

An employee's health records are confidential. Disclosure of information about the employee's HIV status within the hospital community is a serious breach of confidentiality. Employers must provide a system for keeping confidential any health information about their employees, including testing for HIV.

Evaluation of an employee's performance is likewise confidential. If an employee refuses to care for a client with HIV and is counseled or disciplined as a result, the health care agency has an obligation to keep the refusal confidential. Of course, if the employee discloses the refusal, any breach of confidentiality by the employer, while still not ethical, loses its impact and diminishes the legal importance of the breach.

Nondiscriminatory
Employment Opportunities

An employee who is HIV positive should be able to count on the same initial employment opportunities and the same chances for advancement as any other employee. An employer can assess the current health status of a potential employee to determine the person's ability to carry out the requirements of the job. However, if an employer engages in predictive screening—that is, trying to predict who will be capable of performing in the future—the legal risk to the employer increases (Rothstein, 1987).

Case law in this area is developing. For this reason an employing agency may prefer not to know the HIV status of its employees. Lack of knowledge would protect the agency from charges of discrimination based on HIV status.

Assistance with Stress Management

Health care providers have always been subject to unusual job-related stress, but issues surrounding HIV infection have added additional emotional stress as providers care for a group of primarily young people who frequently suffer a great deal before they die. It is also stressful to assist the families and lovers of very sick and dying patients.

In addition to stresses from caring for patients and families, today's care givers must be constantly alert to protect themselves from a very serious infectious disease. It can be expected that they will experience intense job-related stress.

Although health care agencies are not legally required to provide workers with help for stress management, some agencies have accepted an ethical responsibility in this area. These organizations provide a variety of services, including individual and group counseling and education in stress management.

OBLIGATIONS TO PATIENTS

The agency and its employees are responsible to the patient in a variety of ways, including the assignment of rooms, visiting privileges, protection of confidential information, and protection against infection.

If a patient believes that a health care provider has not met acceptable standards, the patient may institute legal action for negligence or malpractice, abandonment, or intentional infliction of emotional distress. In some jurisdictions the patient may sue on the basis of violation of existing state or local statutes, or of the federal statute prohibiting discrimination against a handicapped person. The Department of Health and Human Services, Office of Civil Rights, may be called upon for assistance if a patient believes his or her rights are violated. See Chapter 4 for further discussion of legal issues.

High-Quality Care

The first obligation of a health care agency is to provide the same (presumably high) quality of care to all patients. The agency should carefully monitor and audit quality of care to identify employees who may be giving HIV-positive patients substandard care and should sanction employees accordingly. Quality is often measured by assessing employee compliance with standards such as adherence to infection-control guidelines and policies about treatment of confidential information. The employer can also note whether patients are clean and comfortable, and whether they are receiving treatments and medicines as ordered.

Room Assignment

Sharing a room with a patient who is HIV positive does not present a danger to the HIV-negative patient unless the positive patient also has an airborne infection such as streptococcus or active pulmonary tuberculosis. These infections are relatively rare in HIV-positive patients. A more serious concern would be to protect a person with a damaged immune system from the infections of other patients and staff.

Designation of Acceptable Visitors

Many hospitals have found it necessary to restrict visits to critically ill patients in some way, while others have found ways to manage care with few restrictions on visits. Restrictions have generally allowed entrance only to "family members" and excluded persons not considered part of the patient's immediate family. For many AIDS patients, however, the person they want most to be with as death approaches is not someone in their publicly defined family group.

Hospitals need to redefine family. In 1983, Cliff Morrison, when he was head nurse on the AIDS ward at San Francisco General Hospital, allowed all patients to designate who would have visiting privileges. He believed that it should be the right of the patients themselves to define their families (Shilts, 1987, p. 395).

Confidentiality

Most agencies have adopted universal guidelines for infection prevention so that all patients are treated the same. According to these guidelines, disclosure of information about HIV status is only appropriate when the information is essential to professionals in planning patient care.

Confidentiality of information does not end with death. In state law, however, there is a growing trend to provide information about HIV status to funeral home directors (Rowe & Ryan, 1987, pp. 4–20). These laws may specify the conditions, if any, under which information may be transmitted to a third party.

Protection Against Infection

One of the major reasons to use universal precautions is to protect everyone—patient and provider alike—from infection. Patients who see infection precautions used in all situations will be less likely to blame a health care provider or facility in the event of infection. Previously high rates of hospital-acquired infection should decrease as these guidelines become standard operating procedure in health care agencies.

BIBLIOGRAPHY

American Hospital Association (1987–88). AIDS/HIV infection: Recommendations for health care practices and public policy. AHA Report, p. vii. Chicago: American Hospital Association.

Centers for Disease Control (June 24, 1988). Update: Universal precautions. *Morbidity and Mortality Weekly Report*, p. 378.

Rothstein, M. (1987). Screening workers for AIDS. In H. Dalton, & S. Burris (eds.), AIDS and the Law: A Guide for the Public, p. 128. New Haven: Yale University Press.

Rowe, M., & C. Ryan (October 1987). AIDS, a Public Health Challenge: State Issues, Policies and Programs. Vol. 1. Assessing the Problem. Washington, DC: U.S. Department of Health and Human Services.

Shilts, R. (1987). And the Band Played On: Politics, People and the AIDS Epidemic. New York: St. Martins Press.

U.S. Department of Labor/Department of Health and Human Services (October 30, 1987). Joint advisory notice. HBV/HIV. *Federal Register,* 52:41818–41824.

U.S. Department of Labor, Occupational Safety and Health Administration (August, 1988). Instruction CPL 2-2.44A: Enforcement procedures for occupational exposure to hepatitis B virus (HBV) and human immunodeficiency virus (HIV). Washington, DC: U.S. Department of Labor.

7

QUESTIONS
AND ANSWERS

The purpose of this chapter is to help the health care provider answer common questions that colleagues, patients, and the public ask about AIDS and human immunodeficiency virus (HIV) infection.

THE DISEASE: DIAGNOSIS,
TRANSMISSION, AND PREVENTION

Is HIV infection a sexually transmitted disease?

Yes, predominantly, but not exclusively.

Is HIV infection contagious?

A disease is designated contagious when it is transmitted easily through the air, as with measles. HIV is not casually transmitted and is generally not considered contagious by public health officials.

How does the body protect itself against infection?

The first line of defense against infection in humans is intact skin and mucous membrane; secretions of mucous membranes in the mouth, respiratory tract, stomach, eyes, and vagina also offer some protection. Once a pathogen has entered the body, protection is afforded by special cells and by antibodies produced specifically to combat the invading organism.

How does HIV enter the body?

HIV enters the blood of an uninfected person in the blood, semen, or vaginal fluid of an infected person.

What makes HIV infection so deadly?

The especially devastating effect of HIV in humans is related to the fact that the white blood cell or lymphocyte this virus uses to reproduce is the very cell the body needs to direct an attack on the virus—the T helper cell.

Are there any "warning signs" that predict that an HIV carrier is going to become sick?

Before symptoms of HIV infection appear, the progress of the infection can be detected through determining the numbers and ratios of certain critical white blood cells.

Can people be vaccinated against HIV infection?

Owing to the special nature of this deadly virus, scientists agree that an effective vaccine is still many years away.

How is HIV infection treated?

At present, the only treatment once HIV has entered the body is the administration of chemicals that prevent further multiplication of the virus.

What is an "opportunistic" infection?

An opportunistic infection is caused by a pathogen that has taken the opportunity to invade the body of a person with a depressed immune system. These pathogens, in a healthy person, would not cause debilitating disease because they would be destroyed by an intact immune system.

If viruses are so tiny, how do we know they won't go through latex gloves?

Water molecules are smaller than viruses. If water won't go through latex gloves, then neither will HIV.

If HIV is found in tears, why does the CDC say it probably can't be transmitted that way?

Although small amounts of virus are found in tears, the family members of persons with HIV infection who have had close contact for many years have not become positive.

Why does the CDC say that HIV is not likely to be transmitted by human bites?

Saliva has not been implicated in the transmission of this virus. The usual first-aid measures for human bites should be followed. These include:

- Milk the bite wound to make it bleed.
- Wash the area thoroughly with soap and water.
- Seek medical attention.

Why can't scientists tell us for sure what is true? Why do they insist on saying, "Up to this point, this is what we know"?

Science is based on looking at what *has* happened and predicting, based on experience, what *will* happen. AIDS has only been known since 1981, and information is still coming in. There are certain things about the disease, however, such as how the virus is transmitted, that scientists consider facts.

How do I know if my sexual partner has the disease?

You don't know, and your partner may not know either. Unless you are in a long-term monogamous relationship, you should practice behaviors that are not likely to transmit the disease.

Can you get AIDS from giving blood?

No. Needles and other equipment used by the Red Cross to collect blood are sterile.

If I received a blood transfusion before March 1985, should I worry about AIDS? Should I be tested?

Check with the physician who treated you at that time. If HIV was not prevalent in your area, or if you received a limited number of units of blood, your doctor may advise that the risk was small and may not recommend the test. If you received a transfusion in an area of the country that had a high prevalence of HIV infection shortly before March 1985, your physician may recommend testing.

Can you catch HIV from cats?

No. You cannot catch HIV from any animal or from insect bites.

What is AIDS?

AIDS (acquired immune deficiency syndrome) is an acquired illness of the immune system that reduces the body's ability to fight certain types of infection and cancers.

What causes AIDS?

The human immunodeficiency virus (HIV).

How is HIV infection transmitted?

HIV infection is transmitted through intimate sexual contact, through direct exposure to infected blood or blood products, or from an infected woman to her child before or during birth or through infected breast milk.

What are the symptoms of AIDS?

Symptoms of AIDS include:

- Loss of appetite and unexplained weight loss of more than 10 pounds in 2 months.
- Swollen glands in the neck, armpits, or groin
- Leg weakness or pain
- Unexplained fever lasting more than a week
- Night sweating, often profuse
- Persistent unexplained diarrhea
- Dry cough
- White spots or unusual blemishes in the mouth and throat (candidiasis)
- Painful blisters along the course of a nerve (shingles)
- Painless purple spots on the skin
- Progressive mental deterioration
- Loss of vision and hearing

Is HIV found in sperm?

No. The virus is not found in sperm, but it is found in semen, which contains not only sperm but many white blood cells. The fact that sperm is also present in semen is not important to the transmission of the virus.

Which sexual behaviors can transmit HIV?

The following sexual behaviors can transmit the virus:

- Rectal intercourse, especially if preceded by fisting (inserting a hand or fist into the rectum)
- Sharing needles for intravenous injections
- Vaginal intercourse
- Oral sex
- Deep kissing
- Rimming (anal to mouth contact)
- Sharing dildos or other objects that are inserted into body openings
- Douching or using enemas before or after sex, which can weaken the body's natural defenses against infection.

Which sexual behaviors do not transmit HIV?

The following sexual behaviors do not transmit HIV:

- Talking sexy
- Touching (with no exchange of semen, vaginal fluid, or blood). Gloves may be used. Types of touch may include:
    Hugging
    Stroking
    Cuddling
    Caressing
    Massaging
    Wrestling
    Masturbation
    Kissing (dry)

How do people prevent infection during sexual intercourse?

Having sexual intercourse—vaginal, oral, or rectal—with an infected person is dangerous. Protection through use of a latex condom, latex gloves, or latex oral dam is a good idea.

Does spermicidal jelly kill HIV?

Use of a spermicidal jelly containing nonoxynol-9 for vaginal or rectal intercourse may help to kill the virus.

Do condoms always prevent infection?

No. Condoms sometimes break, especially during rectal sex, which is more traumatic to mucous membranes than is vaginal intercourse. Also, semen or vaginal fluids can be shared, even when condoms are used and remain intact. However, condoms can help to prevent infection if they are used properly.

How should you choose and care for a condom?

- Use latex condoms only. So-called natural membrane condoms are not effective against viral infection.
- Condoms should be stored in a cool, dry place out of direct sunlight.
- Use only condoms that show no sign of damage. A damaged condom may be brittle or discolored.

How do you put a condom on?

- Wash genital area with soap and water.
- Put on condom before any genital contact.
- Place a drop of spermicidal jelly, cream, or foam inside the rolled condom. Do not get lubricant on the shaft of the penis.
- Hold the tip of the condom and unroll it onto the erect penis.
- Leave a space at the tip for collection of semen.
- Be careful not to puncture the condom with fingernails.
- Assure that no air is trapped in the tip of the condom.
- Wear two condoms whenever possible.

How do you lubricate the condom?

Lubricate a condom in the following manner:

- Use water-based lubricants such as KY jelly.
- Do not use petroleum-based or oil-based lubricants such as Vaseline, cooking oil, hair grease, shortening, and lotions. These may weaken the latex and cause failure of the condom.
- Lubrication with a spermicidal jelly containing nonoxynol-9 may provide some added protection.
- Use a small amount of lubricant inside and more lubricant outside the condom.

How do you make sure no semen touches a sex partner?

Make sure no semen touches the partner by following these precautions:

- Withdrawal before climax is the safest practice.
- If a condom breaks during intercourse, withdraw immediately and put on a new condom before continuing sexual activity.
- After ejaculation, take care that the condom does not slip off the penis before withdrawal. To do this, hold the condom firmly and withdraw while the penis is still erect.
- Remove the condom carefully, well away from partner's genital area.
- Discard immediately in a plastic-lined garbage can or bag.
- Do not reuse condoms.
- Wash hands with soap and water after discarding condom.

What precautions should IV drug users take with needles?

IV drug users who are not yet in treatment programs should take the following precautions to prevent HIV infection:

- Don't go to shooting galleries.
- Don't rent works.
- Use clean equipment, and don't let anyone else use it. Some needles sold on the street may be packaged as "new" but are actually dirty needles that have been rebagged.
- Needles may be cleaned in the following manner:
    Works should be cleaned immediately before use, even if they were cleaned previously.
    Attach the needle to the syringe.
    Place some full-strength bleach in a cup.
    Draw up a full syringe of bleach, then squirt this into a sink, commode, or garbage can. Repeat once.
    Place some water in a cup.
    Draw up a full syringe of water, then squirt this into a sink, commode, or garbage can. Repeat once.
    Do not inject bleach.

Why do hospital personnel wear gloves when they draw blood? Do they think I have AIDS?

No. Hospital personnel generally wear gloves to avoid transmitting infection when they risk coming into contact with anyone's blood.

If the tests for HIV are not presently identifying all infected persons, isn't the blood in blood banks unsafe?

Although there is a small chance that infected blood may "get through" the extensive testing process, this risk is relatively slight. Scientists are improving the tests used so that we may be even more sure that the blood supply is not contaminated.

PROTECTING YOURSELF
AND YOUR PATIENTS

How can a health care provider know which patients have HIV and which patients do not?

There is no way to know this with certainty. Therefore the health care provider must act as if the blood of every person is infected and therefore infectious.

What does the term "universal precautions" mean?

This term refers to the system of infection control advocated by the CDC and by the American Hospital Association. It is based on the assumption that all blood, and certain body fluids, may be infectious.

Aren't all body fluids considered infectious for HIV?

No. Body fluids that are not considered to be infectious for HIV, unless they contain visible blood, include: feces, nasal secretions, sputum, sweat, tears, urine, and vomitus. A health care provider may choose to wear gloves, however, when contact with any of these substances is likely, for esthetic reasons or to prevent transfer of infectious organisms by routes other than blood.

What is the most important measure to take in preventing transmission of HIV?

The two most important measures to take are consistent handwashing and care when handling needles and other sharp instruments.

Are laboratory specimens dangerous?

Yes. Laboratory specimens of blood and other body fluids containing visible blood are dangerous. They should be handled with special care according to hospital protocol.

Should I provide direct patient care if I have sores on my hands?

No. With open sores your chances of receiving or transmitting a pathogen are increased. If open areas are small, a physician may decide that you may work safely by using latex gloves.

Is it safe for a pregnant worker to care for a person who is infected with HIV?

The same precautions that protect all health care providers protect a pregnant woman. Some organizations will not assign a pregnant worker to a patient who is actively excreting cytomegalovirus (CMV) because this virus can harm a fetus.

What should be done if blood or body fluid containing blood is spilled?

The spill should be removed with latex-gloved hands and paper towels and the residue wiped up with a bleach and water solution. The solution most frequently recommended is a 1:10 household bleach solution, which is prepared by mixing nine parts water with one part bleach. To be effective, this solution must be mixed daily.

How can inhalation of bleach fumes be avoided?

Bleach solution may be safely mixed by standing well away from the container and pouring the water into the container before pouring in the bleach.

What other precautions should be taken with bleach solution?

Never mix bleach solution with any product containing ammonia.

Why should needles not be recapped?

Recapping needles after use frequently results in needle-stick injury. The CDC guidelines state, "Do not recap used needles by hand; do not remove used needles from disposable syringes by hand; and do not bend, break or otherwise manipulate used needles by hand" (Centers for Disease Control, June 24, 1988).

What should I do if I am accidentally stuck with a used needle or otherwise exposed to a patient's blood?

Most health care organizations have a protocol to follow if an employee has a needle-stick or other exposure to a patient's blood. If such a protocol is not available to you, you may call the CDC Hospital Infections Program at (404) 639-1644 for advice.

What precautions should be taken with equipment used to assess vital signs?

If blood pressure cuffs become contaminated with blood, the outer cuff should be removed and washed and the rubber bladder should be cleaned with alcohol or as directed by the manufacturer. The stethoscope head should be cleaned with alcohol between patients. Temperature should be taken with the patient's personal thermometer when possible; otherwise, use a thermometer with a disposable cover.

What is the appropriate first-aid for accidental ingestion of bleach solution?

The following first-aid measures should be followed:

- Do not induce vomiting.
- Administer milk or water to dilute the solution and to coat the esophagus.
- Try to prevent coughing, in order to avoid aspiration of the chemical.
- Notify the local poison control center immediately, and report the amount and strength of the ingested solution. The center will advise on further treatment.

What special precautions must be taken with the dishes of people who are HIV positive?

No special precautions are necessary. Dishwashing by hand in hot, soapy water will kill HIV.

How should the linens and clothing of HIV-positive persons be handled?

Bloody linens of all persons should be handled with gloves, bagged near the patient's bed, and transported in leak-proof bags. Linens may be safely machine washed with detergent and warm or hot water at the regular cycle.

THE TEST

Why do blood tests for HIV look for HIV antibodies rather than for the virus itself?

Blood is not tested directly for the virus because the equipment and expertise necessary to test directly are presently available in only a few sophisticated laboratories in the United States.

What tests are used to find out if a person's blood is infected?

A series of three tests using one small sample of blood is presently used to identify antibody to HIV. This series consists of two enzyme-linked immunoabsorbent assays (ELISA) and a Western blot or immunofluorescent assay. Only when the result of the entire series is positive is the person considered HIV positive. HIV-positive blood is presumed to be infected and infectious.

What does "seroconversion" mean?

The process of going from a *seronegative* state (no HIV antibodies found in the serum) to a *seropositive* state (HIV antibodies present) is called *seroconversion.*

How long does seroconversion take?

Although infection occurs as soon as the virus enters the body, seroconversion takes several weeks to several months, or longer.

What is the *incubation period* for AIDS?

The incubation period is the length of time between infection (when the virus first entered the blood) and diagnosis. The incubation period for AIDS is presently considered to be between 2 and 15 years (Mann *et al.*, 1988).

Is the antibody test accurate?

The test has been found to be *very accurate* in screening blood donations and in testing organs and semen that are to be donated; the test is also *very accurate* when used in high-risk groups in which many people have the virus. On the other hand, one ELISA without follow-up tests could be quite *inaccurate* (it could give many false-positive results) when used in the general population.

What does a *true-positive* antibody test mean?

A true-positive antibody test result (on the confirming Western blot test) means that the person is infected with the virus and may become sick at some time in the future. The person must assume that he or she can infect others by exchange of blood, semen, or vaginal fluid.

What does a *true-negative* test mean?

Negative test results may have several interpretations. The person may not be infected, or the person may be in the early stage of developing an immune response, or the person may have some condition that prevents the immune system from developing antibodies. A true-negative result means the person is not infected.

What does the antibody test not reveal?

Although the test is generally quite accurate in identifying blood that is infected with HIV, the test will not predict which people will become sick with AIDS or with any of the debilitating conditions associated with HIV infection. Also, the test will not identify people who are infected but for one reason or another are not producing antibodies to the virus.

Is it advisable to use a home testing kit for HIV?

No. Accuracy cannot be assured in a home test, and the necessary counseling about the possible meanings of test results is not available at home.

What information should be provided to a person before he or she consents to be tested for HIV?

Patients should be given information about the medical and social meaning of test results and about the various settings in which they may be tested. Only with such information can a person make a meaningful decision to submit to the test.

What part does counseling play in HIV-antibody testing?

Counseling that includes essential information about HIV infection and transmission is considered by many public health officials as the most important part of HIV-antibody testing. This is because such counseling may lead to change in behavior.

Why not test all hospitalized patients?

Testing all people who enter the hospital for HIV would be a major expense for very little benefit. It is easier and far more effective in preventing transfer of disease organisms to implement HIV infection-control practices as standard operating procedure rather than to use those practices only for patients known to be HIV positive. Also, people have the right to choose to not submit to a test.

What is an *anonymous* test site?

In an anonymous test site no names or other personally identifying data are collected, although basic information such as race and age may be gathered. Numbers are used to match test results with clients.

What is a *counseling and testing* site?

The CDC has funded the Counseling and Testing Site (CTS) Program so that people can receive anonymous or confidential testing. Tests are provided at low or no cost. The sites are generally managed by the state, county, or local departments of health.

SOCIAL, ETHICAL, AND
LEGAL ISSUES

What is homophobia?

Homophobia, or the fear of homosexuals, is a fear of gays and lesbians. This fear has led to a variety of discriminatory acts against individuals thought to be members of these groups.

Isn't AIDS a disease that affects mainly gay white males?

Although AIDS has been presented in the U.S. media as a disease of gay white males, this perception is not accurate. The disease is also prevalent in the black and Latino communities, in heterosexual men, and among women and children.

What is the difference between a crime and a tort?

A crime is an action committed against *society* (the state); a tort is an action against an *individual*. Conviction of a crime results in a fine or imprisonment; conviction of a tort results in payment of money for damages to the injured person.

Doesn't a health care provider have a right to know if a particular patient is HIV positive?

No. The CDC has issued guidelines known as "universal precautions" requiring health care providers to treat all blood as if it were infected. If providers follow these guidelines neither the provider nor the patient need know the HIV status of the other.

Can a nursing assistant, ward clerk, or housekeeper be sued for malpractice?

No. Only those health care providers who practice under a professional license are subject to a malpractice action. Others may be prosecuted for negligence—a breach of duty owed by any reasonable person.

What is malpractice?

Malpractice is professional negligence. It is prosecuted under civil (tort) law. Malpractice acknowledges that the duty of a licensed professional to a patient is a higher duty than the duty of one layperson to another.

What is meant by "breach of duty" in a malpractice case?

Breach of duty may refer to something the professional *did* but should not have done or to something the professional *did not do* but should have done.

Can an institution other than a court of law discipline a health care professional?

Professional licensing boards can remove members' licenses for breach of ethics (breach of confidentiality or refusal to provide care).

Don't I have a right to know if my child is going to school with a child who is carrying HIV?

No. You may *want* to know, but information about a person's medical history is private. Since HIV is not transmitted casually, there is no reason to make a carrier's history public.

Don't I have a right to know if my child's college roommate is infected with the AIDS virus?

No. All college students should be provided with information on how to stay healthy—that is, on behaviors to avoid to prevent HIV infection.

Can a hospital test my blood for HIV without my permission?

Some hospitals may do it, although testing without informed consent is a violation of your rights. Always ask what tests will be performed on your blood.

COMMUNITY RESOURCES

Who holds the primary responsibility for controlling the AIDS epidemic in the United States?

Although the federal government has accepted some general responsibilities related to study of the epidemic and care for affected persons, controlling the AIDS epidemic is at present primarily a state and local responsibility.

What is a community AIDS task force?

An AIDS task force is a group of individuals who take on the responsibility for managing the social, medical, educational, and legal problems presented by this disease in a local community. Such a group complements the systems of medical, psychological, and social networks already in place.

THE OBLIGATIONS OF EMPLOYERS

What are the obligations of the employer to the health care provider with respect to AIDS?

The employer has a duty to provide all employees with information about protection against AIDS, policies consistent with accepted standards, protective gear and equipment to use in patient care, procedures to be followed when a potentially infectious incident has occurred on the job, assurance that an employee's health records are confidential, and nondiscriminatory employment.

What obligations does the health care agency have to a patient?

The agency and its employees are responsible to the patient in a variety of ways, including the assignment of rooms, decisions about who may visit and when, protection of confidential information, and protection against transmission of infection in the hospital through careless acts of employees.

BIBLIOGRAPHY

Centers for Disease Control (June 24, 1988). Update: Universal precautions. *Morbidity and Mortality Weekly Report*, p. 378.

Rowe, M., & C. Ryan (1987). AIDS: A Public Health Challenge. Vol. 1. Assessing the Problem, pp. 2–37. Washington, DC: U.S. Department of Health and Human Services.

Mann, D. L., C. Murray, R. Yarchoan, W. Blattner, & J. J. Goedert (1988). HLA antigen frequencies in HIV-1 seropositive disease-free individuals and patients with AIDS. *Journal of Acquired Immune Deficiency Syndromes*, 1(1):13–17.

APPENDIX:
AIDS-RELATED DISEASES
(OPPORTUNISTIC INFECTIONS)

PROTOZOAN INFECTIONS

Pneumocystis carinii *pneumonia (PCP).* The most common opportunistic infection in patients with AIDS. This type of pneumonia or lung infection is caused by a protozoan commonly present in the environment but normally destroyed in people with healthy immune systems. A person who develops PCP is likely to get the disease again, and the outcome is often fatal. However, new treatment is being developed which shows promise for preventing PCP if treatment is begun early in the progression of HIV disease.

Toxoplasma gondii *encephalitis.* An infection in the brain leading to several different types of neurologic disorders.

Cryptosporidium *enteritis.* Caused by a parasite that lodges in the intestines and causes chronic severe diarrhea. In AIDS the condition lasts longer than 1 month.

Isospora *enteritis.* Another acute form of diarrhea that rarely occurs in healthy adults. In AIDS the condition lasts longer than 1 month.

FUNGAL INFECTIONS

Cryptococcal meningitis. An infection, caused by a fungus, of the membranes surrounding the brain and the spinal cord. This meningitis often causes headache, blurred vision, confusion, depression, agitation, or inappropriate speech. The disease may be fatal.

Oral and esophageal candidiasis. A yeast infection of the mouth and esophagus, common in AIDS patients. It is characterized by white patches, reddened mucous membranes, and discomfort in chewing and swallowing. Oral candidiasis is sometimes called "thrush" or "trench-mouth."

Bronchial pulmonary candidiasis. A very rare form of the yeast-like infection described above that affects the lungs and the air passages.

Disseminated histoplasmosis. A disease mainly caused by inhaling spores from soil contaminated by bird droppings. It causes lesions in the liver, spleen, lymph nodes, lining of the brain and spinal cord, adrenal glands, and bone marrow of a person with a depressed immune system. Systems are related to dysfunction in the organ systems which are primarily infected.

BACTERIAL/VIRAL INFECTIONS

Disseminated mycobacterium avium. This bacterial infection causes chronic and acute lung diseases. It is caused by a different species of the same bacterium that causes tuberculosis in humans.

Chronic mucocutaneous herpes simplex. A type of herpes or ulcer-causing disease that affects areas near the openings of the body. There are presently no cures for the diseases caused by the herpes viruses.

Cytomegalovirus (CMV) infection of organs other than lymph nodes and liver. CMV is related to the herpes family. CMV infections generally produce mild flulike symptoms, including aching, fever, mild sore throat, weakness, and enlarged lymph nodes. In persons whose immune systems are impaired, the symptoms may be far more severe, resulting in hepatitis, mononucleosis, retinitis, or pneumonia. CMV infection in pregnancy may cause birth defects.

CANCERS

Kaposi's sarcoma (KS). A cancer which, before the advent of AIDS, was found rarely in persons under 60 years of age. With KS, tumors usually appear in the walls of the blood vessels, causing painless purple spots to appear on the skin. The tumors may also be internal. When the major organs become involved, death usually occurs.

Primary central nervous system lymphoma. This malignant tumor of the lymph tissue in the central nervous system is found not only in patients with HIV infection, but in others who have a depressed immune response. Symptoms include headache, cranial nerve palsies, seizure disorder, partial paralysis, altered mental status, and personality change. Diagnosis by biopsy is necessary to differentiate this disease from others that may be more successfully treated. Radiation treatment may relieve symptoms.

GLOSSARY

AIDS (acquired immune deficiency syndrome). A fatal disease of the immune system that reduces the body's ability to fight certain types of infection and cancers.

AIDS dementia. A degenerative disorder of the brain and central nervous system caused by HIV infection and leading to progressive deterioration of mental and neurological functions.

Antibody. A protein molecule developed by the body's immune system in response to exposure to a specific foreign agent. A given antibody exactly matches the specific infectious agent much as a key matches a lock.

Antigen. A chemical, recognized as foreign by the body, which triggers an immune response in a host. Bacteria and viruses contain such chemicals.

ARC (AIDS-related complex). An intermediate stage of HIV infection, between infection with the virus and diagnosis of AIDS, characterized by generalized enlargement or tenderness of lymph nodes, fatigue, shortness of breath, cough, night sweats, weight loss, persistent diarrhea, rash, and sores in the mouth. ARC is not recognized by the Centers for Disease Control as a category of HIV infection.

Asymptomatic. Without obvious signs of illness. People who are infected with HIV, as shown by the presence of antibodies in the blood, may show no symptoms of disease.

Contact tracing. Active seeking by public officials of the names or identities of persons who have come in contact with or have been exposed to an infectious disease. These contacts, when found, are notified of their possible exposure to the disease.

ELISA (enzyme-linked immunoabsorbent assay) test. A simple blood test that measures antibodies to HIV proteins. The ELISA was licensed by the Food and Drug Administration in 1985 to screen blood. Because false-positive results are sometimes produced, ELISAs are usually repeated if the first test result is positive. Results of this test generally are available within a few days of the test. If the second result is also positive, a Western blot or immunofluorescent assay (IFA) is performed to confirm the results.

Endemic. Belonging or peculiar to a particular geographic area or defined population. For example, HIV infection is estimated to be present in a large percentage of certain well-defined groups and is now considered to be endemic in those populations.

Epidemic. Occurring in a region, population, or community clearly in excess of what is expected. AIDS has reached epidemic proportions in many U.S. urban centers.

Epidemiology. The study of how a disease or condition is distributed in human populations and what factors influence its distribution. Epidemiologists are concerned with how disease patterns change over time, how disease patterns differ by geographic area, and how the characteristics of individuals influence the disease pattern. The personal characteristics of most interest to epidemiologists include basic demographic facts (age, sex, race, ethnic group), biological factors (different blood characteristics), social and economic factors (income, education, occupation), and personal living habits (smoking, diet).

Exposure. Contact with a pathogen such as HIV in a way that makes it possible to become infected and transmit it.

False-negative test result. A negative test result from a person who in fact carries the disease or condition the test attempted to find.

False-positive test result. A positive test result from a person truly not affected by the disease or condition tested for.

Hemophilia. An inherited condition causing a failure of blood to form clots and leaving the person at risk of severe bleeding. Hemophilia is treated by the infusion of blood-clotting factors prepared by pooling plasma from thousands of blood donors. Clotting factors used today are treated to eliminate HIV contamination; for this reason hemophilia is no longer considered a major risk factor for HIV infection.

Hepatitis.   Inflammation of the liver, often caused by poisoning the liver with alcohol or other chemicals, or by infection with hepatitis A, B, or other hepatitis viruses.

Human immunodeficiency virus (HIV).   The virus that causes crippling damage to the immune system in humans and causes the disease AIDS.

Immune system.   A complex network of organs and cells that allows the body to defend itself against infections and harmful substances.

Immunofluorescence assay (IFA).   Serologic test for detecting or confirming the presence of HIV antibodies.

Incidence.   The number of new cases of something occurring in a specified population over a specified period of time, usually 1 year.

Infectious disease.   An illness that results from development or multiplication of a disease-causing organism. Not all infectious diseases are highly contagious or easily communicable. Although HIV is infectious, it is not easily or casually transmitted.

Informed consent.   Assent to a procedure by a patient who understands the implications of the procedure.

Isolation.   The separation of infected persons from others to prevent the spread of disease between infected and uninfected people.

Latency.   Ability of a pathogen to be present within a cell without reproducing. The herpes viruses, which cause cold sores, shingles, and genital herpes, are viruses that can remain latent in humans until they are stimulated to become active.

Latency period.   The time period during which an infection exists without causing any symptoms or the time period from the point of infection to the development of clinical signs of the disease. Based on current data, the latency period for HIV is estimated to range up to 15 years.

Lesion.   A pathological change in structure of an organ. In AIDS a common change is the skin lesion caused by Kaposi's sarcoma.

Meningitis.   Inflammation of the membranes of the spinal cord or brain.

Morbidity.   Illness. Public health officials study illness through the use of incidence and prevalence statistics.

Opportunistic infection.   A disease that occurs in a person who does not have a healthy immune system. Such a disease does not normally occur in a healthy person, but takes the *opportunity* presented by the damaged immune system to take hold and make the person ill.

Pathogen.   A microorganism that causes disease. Pathogens include bacteria, protozoa, fungi, and viruses.

Phagocytosis.   The process, within the body, of engulfing and destroying foreign material (dust, smoke, oil, bacteria, viruses). This process is accomplished by a special white blood cell, the macrophage.

Predictive value.   The likelihood that the results of a test for a particular condition will correlate with the presence or absence of the condition.

Prevalence.   The number of people in a given population who have a disease, measured at a specific point in time.

Risk factors.   Personal characteristics and behaviors that increase the likelihood that a person will be affected by a given condition. A person is believed to be at particularly high risk of contracting HIV infection if he or she:

• Is or was a sexual partner of an HIV-infected person
• Has shared needles with an HIV-infected drug user

- Has received blood, semen, or body organs donated by an HIV-infected patient
- Is a child born to an HIV-infected mother

Screening.   The process of identifying undetected disease by tests, examinations, or other procedures. Screening usually involves simple, quick procedures that can be applied to large numbers of people. The tests are used to separate apparently well persons who probably have a disease from persons who probably do not.

Sensitivity (of a test).   The ability of a test to identify correctly persons with a disease or condition—that is, to identify the "true positives." Most HIV antibody tests are highly sensitive. However, the sensitivity may vary according to the test manufacturer, the prevalence of HIV infection in the test population, the standards employed by the testing laboratory, and the interpretation of the test results.

Seroconversion.   The change in the test status of a person's blood serum from negative for an antibody to positive. With HIV, seroconversion may take from 3 weeks to 6 months or longer with present tests.

Seronegative.   The status of a person's blood when tests cannot confirm that HIV antibodies are present. Generally, a person's blood is considered to be seronegative if 1) the initial ELISA result is negative; 2) the initial ELISA result is positive but the repeat result is negative; or 3) both ELISA results are positive, but the Western blot result is negative.

Seropositive.   The status of a person's blood when tests confirm that HIV antibodies are present. Generally, a person's blood is considered to be seropositive if the results of a series of two ELISAs and of a confirming Western blot or immunofluorescent assay (IFA) are positive.

Specificity (of a test).   The ability of a test to identify correctly people who do not have a disease or condition. The ELISA is not highly specific for HIV antibody, but the series of tests currently used (two ELISAs and one Western blot) is highly specific.

T lymphocyte (T cell).   A type of white blood cell that is essential to the body's immune system in its fight against infection. T cells help regulate the production of substances called antibodies. T4 lymphocytes are a special subset of T cells that start the body's immune response and help the body protect itself against viruses, bacteria, parasites, tumors, and fungi. The HIV virus interferes with the function of the T4 cells.

Transmission.   Transfer of a disease from one person to another. HIV may be transmitted in three main ways:

- Through intimate, unprotected sexual contact
- Through parenteral (through the skin) exposure
- Through pregnancy and the birth process

True-negative test result.   A negative test result from a person who does not carry the disease or condition the test attempted to find.

True-positive test result.   A positive test result from a person who in fact carries the disease or condition tested for.

Virus.   The smallest known pathogen; it cannot live on its own but must enter a functioning cell to multiply.

Western blot.   This relatively expensive test uses viral proteins that attach to HIV antibodies in the patient's serum. It is used at present to confirm or negate a positive ELISA result. Sometimes the results are indeterminate, and the test must be repeated at a later date.

BIBLIOGRAPHY

BOOKS/PAMPHLETS

American College Health Association (1988). The HIV Antibody Test. 15879 Crabbs Branch Way, Rockville, MD: American College Health Association.

American Nurses' Association (1988). Personal Heroism, Professional Activism: Nursing and the Battle Against AIDS. Kansas City, MO: American Nurses' Association.

Beauchamp, D. E., & J. F. Childress (1979). Principles of Biomedical Ethics. New York: Oxford Press.

Benenson, A. S. (ed.) (1985). Control of Communicable Disease in Man, 14th ed. Washington, DC: American Public Health Association.

CA Nurses' Association (1987). AIDS Resource Manual. 1855 Folsom Street, Suite 670, San Francisco, California 94103: California Nurses' Association.

Carbine, M. E., & P. Lee (1988). AIDS into the '90s: Strategies for an Integrated Response to the AIDS Epidemic. Washington, DC: National AIDS Network.

Corless, I. B., & M. Pittman-Lindeman (1988). AIDS: Principles, Practices & Politics. Washington, DC: Hemisphere Publishing Corporation.

Curtin, L., & M. J. Flaherty (eds.) (1982). Nursing Ethics: Theories and Pragmatics. Bowie, MD: Robert J. Brady Company.

Dalton, H. L., & S. Burris (eds.) (1987). AIDS and the Law: A Guide for the Public. New Haven, CT: Yale University Press.

Davis, M. (1988). Lovers, Doctors & the Law: Your Legal Rights & Responsibilities in Today's Sex-Health Crisis New York: Harper & Row.

De Vita, V. T., S. Hellman, & S. A. Rosenberg (eds.) (1988). AIDS, 2nd ed. Philadelphia: J. B. Lippincott.

Frankena, W. K. (1973). Ethics. Englewood Cliffs, NJ: Prentice-Hall.

Goldstein, E. (ed.) (1983–87). The AIDS Crisis. Social Issues Resources Series, Vol. 1. PO Box 2348, Boca Raton, FL.

Griggs, J. (ed.) (1987). AIDS: Public Policy Dimensions. New York: United Hospital Fund of New York.

Kübler-Ross, E. (1987). AIDS: The Ultimate Challenge. New York: Macmillan.

Langone, J. (1988). AIDS: The Facts. Boston: Little, Brown & Co.

Lewis, A. (1988). Nursing Care of the Person with AIDS/ARC. Rockville, MD: Aspen.

Malloy, C., & J. Hartshorn (1989). Acute Care Nursing in the Home: A Holistic Approach. Philadelphia: J. B. Lippincott.

Mass, L. (1988). Medical Answers About AIDS. New York: Gay Men's Health Crisis.

National AIDS Network (1988). NAN Directory of AIDS Education and Service Organizations. Washington, DC: National AIDS Network.

Nilsson, L. (1987). The Body Victorious. New York: Delacorte Press.

Rowe, M., & C. Ryan (October, 1987). AIDS: A Public Health Challenge, Vols. 1, 2, & 3. Washington, DC: U.S. Department of Health and Human Services.

Ruskin, C. (1988). The Quilt. New York: Pocket Books.

Senak, M. S. (1988). Legal Answers About AIDS. New York: Gay Men's Health Crisis.

Shilts, R. (1987). And the Band Played On: Politics, People and the AIDS Epidemic. New York: St. Martins Press.

Veatch, R. M., & S. T. Fry (1987). Case Studies in Nursing Ethics. Philadelphia: J. B. Lippincott.

West, K. H. (1987). Infectious Disease Handbook for Emergency Care Personnel. Philadelphia: J. B. Lippincott.

JOURNAL AND NEWSPAPER ARTICLES

Altman, L. K. (August 14, 1988). New studies point to fungus as leading to AIDS deaths. *New York Times*.

American Medical Association Council on Ethical and Judicial Affairs (1988). Ethical issues involved in the growing AIDS crisis. *Journal of the American Medical Association, 259*(9):1360–1361.

Arno, P. S. (1986). AIDS: A balancing act of resources. *Business and Health 4*(2):20–24.

Barrick, B. (November, 1988). Caring for AIDS patients: A challenge you can meet. *Nursing 88*:50–59.

Barrick, B. (1988). The willingness of nursing personnel to care for patients with acquired immune deficiency syndrome: A survey study and recommendations. *Journal of Professional Nursing, 4*(5), 366–372.

Beimiller, L. (December 4, 1985). The last weeks of an AIDS patient: A friend remembers. *The Chronicle of Higher Education, 1*:34–36.

Brown, V. L., & J. W. Brown (1988). The third international conference on AIDS: Risk of AIDS in healthcare workers. *Nursing Management, 19*(3):33–35.

Council on Ethical and Judicial Affairs (1988). Ethical issues involved in the growing AIDS crisis. *Journal of the American Medical Association, 259*(9):1360.

Flaskerud, J. H. (1987). AIDS: Implications for mental health nurses. *Journal of Psychosocial Nursing and Mental Health Services, 25*(12):4–6.

Flaskerud, J. H. (1987). AIDS: Neuropsychiatric complications. *Journal of Psychosocial Nursing and Mental Health Services, 25*(12):17–20.

Flaskerud, J. H. (1987). AIDS: Psychosocial aspects. *Journal of Psychosocial Nursing and Mental Health Services, 25*(12):8–16.

Gallo, R., & L. Montagnier (1988). AIDS in 1988. *Scientific American, 259*(4):40–48.

Gerberding, J. L., & D. K. Henderson (1987). Design of rational infection control policies for human immunodeficiency virus infection. *The Journal of Infectious Diseases, 156*(6):861–864.

Graham, L., & J. A. Cates (1987). AIDS: Developing a primary health care task force. *Journal of Psychosocial Nursing and Mental Health Services, 5255*(12): 21–25.

Henderson, D. K. (September/October 1988). AIDS and the health-care worker: Management of human immunodeficiency virus infection in the health-care setting. *AIDS Updates, 1*(1):3–4.

House rejects bid to require disclosure to AIDS spouses (September 17, 1988). *New York Times.*

Jaret, P. (1986). Our immune system: The wars within. *National Geographic, 169*(6):702–734.

Levine, M. (1977). Nursing ethics and the ethical nurse. *American Journal of Nursing, 77*(5):846.

Lewis, L. (1988). Hospitals struggle with HIV antibody testing: Three hospitals have formal policies. *AIDS Patient Care, 2*(4):12–14.

Mann, D. L., C. Murray, R. Yarchoan, W. Blattner, & J. J. Goedert (1988). HLA antigen frequencies in HIV-1 seropositive disease-free individuals and patients with AIDS. *Journal of Acquired Immune Deficiency Syndromes, 1*(1):13–17.

Mann, J. M., J. Chin, P. Piot, & T. Quinn (1988). The international epidemiology of AIDS. *Scientific American, 259*(4):82–89.

Matthews, T. J., & D. P. Bolognesi (1988). AIDS vaccines. *Scientific American, 259*(4):120–127.

Mays, V. M., & S. D. Cochran (1987). Acquired immune deficiency syndrome and black Americans: Special psychological issues. *Public Health Reports, 102*(2):224–231.

Right to bar treatment by any with AIDS virus weighed. September 16, 1988. *New York Times.*

Rogers, M. F., & W. W. Williams (1987). AIDS in blacks and Hispanics: Implications for prevention. *Issues in Science and Technology, 3*(3):89–94.

Schobel, D. A. (1988). Management's responsibility to deal effectively with the risk of HIV exposure for healthcare workers. *Nursing Management, 19*(3):38–42.

Sears, C. (1988). Volunteers: How to get them, train them, and keep them. *AIDS Patient Care, 2*(4):18–20.

Sedaka, S. D., & M. O'Reilly (1986). The financial implications of AIDS. *Caring, V*(6):38–46.

Selik, R. M., K. G. Catro, & M. Pappaioanou (1988). Racial/ethnic differences in the risk of AIDS in the United States. *American Journal of Public Health, 78*(12):1539–1545.

Weber, J. N., & R. A. Weiss (1988). HIV infection: The cellular picture. *Scientific American, 259*(4):100–109.

Wertz, D. C., J. R. Sorenson, L. Liebling, L. Kessler, & T. C. Heeren (1987). Knowledge and attitudes of AIDS health care providers before and after education programs. *Public Health Reports, 102*(3):248–254.

Wiley, K., & J. Grohar (May/June 1988). Human immunodeficiency virus and precautions for obstetric, gynecologic and neonatal nurses. *Journal of Obstetric, Gynecologic, and Neonatal Nursing, 17*(3):165–168.

Wing, K. R. (1986). Constitutional protection of sexual privacy in the 1980's: What is big brother doing in the bedroom? *American Journal of Public Health, 6*(2):201–204.

Wormser, G. P., C. Joline, S. L. Sivak, & A. A. Zalmen (1988). Human immunodeficiency virus infections: Considerations for health care workers. *Bulletin of the New York Academy of Medicine, 64*(3):203–215.

Yarchoan, R., H. Mitsuya, & S. Broder (1988). AIDS therapies. *Scientific American, 259*(4):110–119.

REPORTS AND POLICY STATEMENTS

American College Health Association (1985). General statement of institutional response to AIDS. 15879 Crabbs Branch Way, Rockville, MD: American College Health Association.

American College Health Association (1985). What everyone should know. 15879 Crabbs Branch Way, Rockville, MD: American College Health Association.

American Hospital Association (1987–88). AIDS/HIV infection: Recommendations for health care practices and public policy. AHA Report. Chicago: American Hospital Association.

American Hospital Association (July, 1988). AIDS memo-
    randum #3: HIV testing and informed consent. AIDS
    issues update. Chicago: American Hospital Association.
American Medical Association (1980). Principles of medi-
    cal ethics. Chicago: American Medical Association.
American Medical Association Council on Ethical and
    Judicial Affairs (1986). Statement on AIDS. Chicago:
    American Medical Association.
American Nurses' Association (1976). Code for nurses.
    Kansas City: American Nurses' Association.
Bureau of National Affairs (1986). AIDS in the workplace:
    Resource material. 9435 Key West Avenue, Rockville,
    MD 20850: Bureau of National Affairs.
Centers for Disease Control (February 7, 1986). Apparent
    transmission of human T-lymphotropic virus type III/
    lymphadenopathy-assocated virus from a child to a
    mother providing health care. Morbidity and Mortality
    Weekly Report: 76–79.
Centers for Disease Control (April 24, 1987). Classifica-
    tion system for human immunodeficiency virus (HIV)
    infection in children under 13 years of age. Morbidity
    and Mortality Weekly Report: 225–230; 235.
Centers for Disease Control (March 11, 1988). Condoms
    for prevention of sexually transmitted diseases. Morbid-
    ity and Mortality Weekly Report: 133–137.
Centers for Disease Control (August 30, 1985). Educa-
    tion and foster care of children infected with human
    T-lymphotropic virus type III/lymphadenopathy-
    associated virus. Morbidity and Mortality Weekly Re-
    port: 517–519.
Centers for Disease Control (1988). Facts about AIDS.
    Washington, DC: U.S. Department of Health and Hu-
    man Services.
Centers for Disease Control (1987). Guidelines for AIDS
    prevention program operations. Washington, DC: U.S.
    Department of Health and Human Services.
Centers for Disease Control (July 1, 1988). Partner notifi-
    cation for preventing human immunodeficiency virus
    (HIV) infection—Colorado, Idaho, South Carolina, Vir-
    ginia. Morbidity and Mortality Weekly Report: 393–396.

Centers for Disease Control (August 14, 1987). Public health service guidelines for counseling and antibody testing to prevent HIV infection and AIDS. Morbidity and Mortality Weekly Report: 509–515.

Centers for Disease Control (September 16, 1988). Quarterly report to the domestic policy council on the prevalence and rate of spread of HIV and AIDS—United States. Morbidity and Mortality Weekly Report: 551–559.

Centers for Disease Control (December 6, 1985). Recommendations for assisting in prevention of perinatal transmission of human T-lymphotropic virus type III/lymphadenopathy-associated virus and acquired immune deficiency syndrome. Morbidity and Mortality Weekly Report: 721–726; 731–732.

Centers for Disease Control (August 21, 1987). Recommendations for prevention of HIV transmission in health-care settings. Morbidity and Mortality Weekly Report (suppl. no. 2S) 35–125.

Centers for Disease Control (October 7, 1988). Transmission of HIV through bone transplantation: Case report and public health recommendations. Morbidity and Mortality Weekly Report: 597–599.

Centers for Disease Control (February 7, 1986). Tuberculosis—United States, 1985—and the possible impact of human T-lymphotropic virus type III/lymphadenopathy-associated virus infection. Morbidity and Mortality Weekly Report: 74–76.

Centers for Disease Control (1988). Understanding AIDS. Washington, DC: U.S. Department of Health and Human Services.

Centers for Disease Control (June 24, 1988). Update: Universal precautions for prevention of transmission of human immunodeficiency virus, hepatitis B virus, and other bloodborne pathogens in health-care settings. Morbidity and Mortality Weekly Report: 377–382; 387–388.

Centers for Disease Control (May 17, 1985). World health organization workshop: Conclusions and recommendations on acquired immunodeficiency syndrome. Morbidity and Mortality Weekly Report: 275–276.

Department of Health and Human Services/Public Health Service (1985). Public health service plan for the prevention and control of acquired immune deficiency syndrome (AIDS). Public Health Reports, 100(5):453–544.

Department of Health and Human Services/Public Health Service (1987). Report of the surgeon general's workshop on children with HIV infection and their families. Washington, DC: U.S. Department of Health and Human Services.

Department of Health and Human Services/Public Health Service (1987). Surgeon general's report on acquired immune deficiency syndrome. Washington, DC: U.S. Department of Health and Human Services.

Department of Labor/Department of Health and Human Services (October 30, 1987). Joint advisory notice: HBV/HIV. Federal Register, 52:41818–41824.

Institute of Medicine, National Academy of Sciences (1986). Confronting AIDS: Directions for public health, health care, and research. Washington, DC: National Academy Press.

Institute of Medicine, National Academy of Sciences (1988). Confronting AIDS: Update 1988. Washington, DC: National Academy Press.

Intragovernmental Task Force (1987). AIDS health care delivery. Washington, DC: U.S. Department of Health and Human Services.

National Institute of Mental Health (1986). Coping with AIDS. Washington, DC: U.S. Department of Health and Human Services.

Occupational Safety and Health Administration, Office of Health Compliance (August, 1988). Instruction CPL 2-2.44A, Enforcement procedures for occupational exposure to hepatitis B virus (HBV) and human immunodeficiency virus (HIV). Washington, DC: U.S. Department of Labor.

INDEX

Note: Page numbers in *italics* indicate illustrations.

Abused women, management
 of, 45–47
Addiction, drug. *See* Drug
 abuse
AIDS. *See also* Human
 immunodeficiency
 virus
 categories of, 9–13
 and confidentiality issues.
  See Confidentiality
 diagnosis of, 6–8
 disease progression in, 6, *7,*
  10–13, *11*
 ethical issues involving, 67,
  111–112
 fears involving, 1, 63–64
 history of, 1
 impact of, 8–9
 legal issues involving,
  67–76, 111–112. *See
  also* Legal issues
 morbidity and mortality in,
  8–9
 opportunistic infections in,
  14–16, 114–116
 overview of, 6–8
 prevention of. *See*
  Preventive measures
 questions and answers
  about, 98–113
 signs and symptoms of, 8, 13
 societal issues involving,
  62–67, 111–112
 transmission categories for,
  9–10
 transmission of, 18–21
  via blood, 20–21

AIDS (*continued*)
 questions and answers
  about, 98–108
 sexual, 19–20
 vaccine for, 6, 16
AIDS hotline, 88–89
AIDS-related complex, 12
AIDS task force, 83–89
American Medical
  Association, ethical
  code of, 67
American Nurses'
  Association Code for
  Licensed Practical
  Nurses, 67, 69
American Nurses'
  Association Code for
  Nurses, 67, 68
Ammonia, and bleach, 31
Animal bites, 100
Anonymous testing, 59–60
Answers, to commonly asked
  questions, 98–113
Antigen-antibody reaction,
  2–3
Antiviral therapy, 17–18
Apparel, protective, 27–28,
  30, 91–92, 104–105
Aprons, 28
ARC (AIDS-related complex),
  12–13
Azidothymidine, 17

Bandages, disposal of, 39
Battered women, management
  of, 45–47

131